# Decision Making in Psychopharmacology

# Decision Making in Psychopharmacology

**Siegfried Kasper** MD

*Professor and Chairman*
*Department of General Psychiatry, University of Vienna, Austria*

**Joseph Zohar** MD

*Associate Professor of Psychiatry and Director of Psychiatry*
*Department and Anxiety and Obsessive Compulsive Clinic*
*Chaim Sheba Medical Center, Tel Hashomer, Israel*

**Dan J. Stein MD,** PhD

*Director, MRC Unit on Anxiety Disorders*
*University of Stellenbosch, Cape Town and*
*University of Florida, Gainesville, USA*

**MARTIN DUNITZ**

© 2002 Martin Dunitz Ltd, a member of the Taylor & Francis group

First published in the United Kingdom in 2002
by Martin Dunitz, Taylor & Francis Group plc, 11 New Fetter Lane, Lo

Tel.: +44 (0) 20 7583 9855
Fax.: +44 (0) 20 7842 2298
E-mail: info@dunitz.co.uk
Website:    http://www.dunitz.co.uk

Although every effort has been made to ensure that all owners of copyright material have
been acknowledged in this publication, we would be glad to acknowledge in subsequent
reprints or editions any omissions brought to our attention.

A CIP record for this book is available from the British Library.

ISBN 1-85317-594-3

Distributed in the USA by Fulfilment Center, Taylor & Francis, 10650 Tobben Drive,
Independence, KY 41051, USA
Toll Free Tel.: +1 800 634 7064
E-mail: taylorandfrancis@thomsonlearning.com

Distributed in Canada by Taylor & Francis, 74 Rolark Drive, Scarborough,
Ontario M1R 4G2, Canada
Toll Free Tel.: +1 877 226 2237
E-mail: tal_fran@istar.ca

Distributed in the rest of the world by Thomson Publishing Services, Cheriton House,
North Way, Andover, Hampshire SP10 5BE, UK
Tel.: +44 (0)1264 332424
E-mail: salesorder.tandf@thomsonpublishingservices.co.uk

Tables 1.1 (page 2), 2.1 (page 14), 3.1 (page 26), 4.1 (page 36), 5.1 (page 50), 6.1 (pages
59 ff), 7.1 (page 70), 8.2 (page 87) are reprinted with permission from the *Diagnostic and
Statistical Manual of Mental Disorders*, Fourth Edition, Text Revision. Washington, DC:
American Psychiatric Association, 2000. © American Psychiatric Association, 2000.

The cover illustration was drawn by Natalie Weil

Printed and bound in Italy by Printer Trento Srl.

# Contents

Introduction ix

1 Pharmacotherapy of unipolar depression 1
  *Siegfried Kasper and Joseph Zohar*

2 Pharmacotherapy of bipolar disorder 13
  *Siegfried Kasper and Joseph Zohar*

3 Pharmacotherapy of schizophrenia 25
  *Siegfried Kasper and Joseph Zohar*

4 Pharmacotherapy of panic disorder 35
  *Robert MA Hirschfeld, Joseph Zohar and Dan J Stein*

5 Pharmacotherapy of social anxiety disorder 47
  *Joseph Zohar, Siegfried Kasper and Dan J Stein*

6 Pharmacotherapy of post-traumatic stress disorder 57
  *Joseph Zohar, Siegfried Kasper and Dan J Stein*

7 Pharmacotherapy of obsessive-compulsive disorder 69
  *Joseph Zohar, Siegfried Kasper and Dan J Stein*

8 Pharmacotherapy of dementia of the Alzheimer's type 81
  *Franz Müller-Spahn and Siegfried Kasper*

Index 107

*We would like to dedicate this book
to our beloved wives*

## Anita Kasper

*and*

## Rachel Zohar

*and*

## Heather Zar

*who have supported us
so constantly over the years*

# About the authors

**Siegfried Kasper MD** is Professor of Psychiatry and Chairman of the Department of General Psychiatry at the University of Vienna, Austria. He has clinical and research experience in psychiatry, neurology, psychotherapeutics and psychoanalysis from various institutions. Professor Kasper is involved in research programmes in depression, anxiety, psychosis and dementia. He is on the executive committees and advisory boards of several national and international societies. He was President of the 10th ECNP Congress in Vienna in 1997, is involved in projects of the WHO and is an adviser to the European Agency for the Evaluation of Medicinal Products. Professor Kasper is Co-Editor-in-Chief of the *International Journal of Psychiatry in Clinical Practice* and he is on the editorial boards of several other journals. He has written over 650 papers, concentrating on the biological bases of mental disorders and their possible treatment approaches.

**Joseph Zohar MD** is a Director in the Division of Psychiatry at the Chaim Sheba Medical Center, Ramat Gan, Israel and of that institution's Anxiety and Obsessive-Compulsive Clinic and Associate Professor of Psychiatry at the Sackler School of Medicine. He has been elected chairperson of several organizations, including the Anxiety and OCD section of the WPA (World Psychiatric Association) and the International Council on Anxiety and OCD. Professor Zohar was a member of the DSM-IV Obsessive-Compulsive Disorder subcommittee, and he is currently a member of the executive committee of the ECNP and a member of the WHO Expert Advisory Panel on Neuroscience. He has won several awards, including the AE Bennett award in 1986 and the European College of Neuropsychopharmacology award for clinical research.

Professor Zohar is Associate Editor of the *World Journal of Biological Psychiatry*, Editor-in-Chief of the journal *Focus on OCD*, and International Editor of the journal *CNS Spectrums*. He is on the editorial boards of several other journals. He has edited ten books, written two books (on depression and OCD), and is the author of over 200 scientific papers related to pre-clinical and clinical research in psychiatry.

**Dan Stein MD, PhD** is Associate Professor of Psychiatry at the University of Stellenbosch in Cape Town, South Africa, and is Research Associate Professor at the University of Florida in Gainesville, USA. He directs a research unit on anxiety disorders; the Unit is funded by the Medical Research Council (MRC) of South Africa, and focuses on the psychobiology of the anxiety disorders. He also plays an active role in a number of national and international psychiatry organizations. Professor Stein's work has been recognized with a number of honours, including awards from the Anxiety Disorders Association of America, the World Psychiatric Association Section on OCD, and Collegium Internationale Neuropsychopharmacologicum. Professor Stein is on the editorial boards of several journals, including *International Journal of Neuropsychopharmacology, World Journal of Biological Psychiatry,* and *CNS Spectrums*. He has edited several books on anxiety disorders and on cognitive science, and is the author of over 300 papers and chapters.

Parts of this book were written in collaboration with:

Robert MA Hirschfeld MD
*Titus Harris Distinguished Professor*
*Chair, Department of Psychiatry and Behavioral Sciences*
*The University of Texas – Medical Branch, Galveston, USA*

Franz Müller-Spahn MD
*Professor and Medical Director*
*Department of Psychiatry*
*University of Basel, Switzerland*

# Introduction

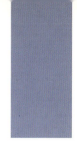

Psychopharmacology is a rapidly advancing field; each year sees the introduction of new agents and the publication of many trials. This book aims to highlight the different available avenues of treatment and to stimulate a discussion about the evaluative process that we, as physicians, use in treating our patients in everyday practice. It is meant to help doctors to reconsider their own opinions and to justify their own treatment recommendations, on the basis of the knowledge available in the literature.

Despite advances in psychopharmacology research, there are many areas of clinical decision making where published evidence is sparse. Our approach in this volume is to differentiate for the reader areas where the evidence is stronger from areas where there is less evidence (see the Table below). We hope that *Decision Making in Psychopharmacology* will provide a tool for assisting the decision-making process in everyday clinical practice.

Each of the chapters follows a specific pattern, which aims to help the reader specify the nature of particular decisions. Decision levels range from applying the treatment of choice (based on several consistent randomized controlled trials), to switching and augmentation strategies, through to other treatment options (for which there may be some controlled data), and on to more experimental approaches. The major diagnostic categories are dealt with, including unipolar depression, bipolar disorder, schizophrenia, panic disorder, post-traumatic stress disorder, social anxiety disorder, obsessive-compulsive disorder and dementia of the Alzheimer's type.

We are aware that algorithms to psychiatric treatment have been criticized as comprising a 'cookbook' approach. However, we believe that a volume such as the present one, which represents an evidence-based 'menu' of possibilities (rather than a single option), can enhance the evaluative process which doctors go through with their patients, allowing an integration of 'clinical wisdom' with current available knowledge. Algorithms cannot replace clinical judgement; our hope is that this volume will help strengthen good clinical practice.

Siegfried Kasper MD
*Professor and Chairman*
*Department of General Psychiatry*
*University of Vienna, Austria*

Joseph Zohar MD
*Director, Psychiatry Department and Anxiety and OCD Clinic*
*Chaim Sheba Medical Centre*
*Tel Hashomer, Israel*

Dan J. Stein MD, PhD
*Director, MRC Unit on Anxiety Disorders*
*University of Stellenbosch, Cape Town, South Africa and*
*University of Florida, Gainesville, USA*

## LEVELS OF EVIDENCE

**Level 1** Intervention supported by consistent randomized controlled trials (green)

**Level 2** Intervention supported by limited controlled data (yellow)

**Level 3** Intervention supported by uncontrolled data (pink)

**Level 4** Interventions that have been found to be ineffective (red)

# Pharmacotherapy of unipolar depression

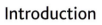

## Introduction

Prior to a treatment decision being made, a firm diagnosis is necessary, establishing that depression is present (major depressive disorder as characterized by DSM-IV or ICD-10), and determining a possible subgroup (Table 1.1). Major depression can be subdivided according to the severity of depression (mild, moderate or severe), by the presence or absence of melancholia and psychotic features, and by a seasonal pattern specifier (fall/winter depression in most cases).[1] Epidemiological data reveal that the lifetime prevalence rate of major depression in the general population is at least 8–10%, although a few studies have indicated that it may even be higher.[2]

Taken together, the overall efficacy of antidepressants is about 60–70%, regardless of pharmacodynamic or pharmacokinetic properties. This means that in about two-thirds of patients the antidepressant chosen first is successful for acute treatment. Nevertheless, the diagnostic subgroups of depression mentioned above, as well as other factors – such as comorbid medical or psychiatric conditions, the presence of suicidality, age or concurrent medication – all contribute to the outcome and can influence the choice of antidepressant.[3,4] Although antidepressants are successful in around two-thirds of patients during short-term treatment, poor tolerability during long-term treatment diminishes the chances that a successful outcome will be maintained.

This volume focuses primarily on pharmacotherapy. Nevertheless, it should be emphasized that pharmacotherapy and psychotherapy do not exclude one another. Indeed, some research suggests that a

***Table 1.1*** *Diagnostic criteria for major depressive episode.*

| DSM-IV criteria for a major depressive disorder, single episode (code 296.2x) |
| --- |
| A. Five (or more) of the following symptoms (as **changes** from previous functioning) occurring nearly every day for 2 weeks; must **include** symptoms of depressed mood and/or loss of interest or pleasure but **exclude** symptoms caused by a general medical condition, or mood-incongruent delusions or hallucinations:<br>• depressed mood most of the day<br>• markedly diminished interest or pleasure in most or all activities most of the day<br>• weight loss or gain (65% body weight/month), or appetite change<br>• insomnia or hypersomnia<br>• psychomotor agitation or retardation<br>• fatigue or loss of energy<br>• feelings of worthlessness or excessive or inappropriate guilt<br>• reduced ability to think or concentrate, or indecisiveness |
| B. Symptoms do not meet criteria for a mixed episode |
| C. Symptoms cause significant impairment in work and social life |
| D. Symptoms not caused by a substance such as a drug or hormone |
| E. Symptoms not better accounted for by bereavement |
| ICD-10 criteria for a depressive episode (category F32) |
| A. The depressive episode should last for at least 2 weeks |
| B. There have been no hypomanic or manic symptoms sufficient to meet the criteria for hypomanic or manic episode (category F30.x) at any time in the individual's life |
| C. Most commonly used exclusion clause: the episode is not attributable to psychoactive substance use (categories F10–F19) or to any organic mental disorder (in the sense of F00–F09) |
| **Somatic syndrome**<br>Some depressive symptoms are widely regarded as having special clinical significance; these are called 'somatic' in the ICD-10. (Terms such as 'biological', 'vital', 'melancholic', and 'endogenomorphic' are used in other classifications.) |

*Table 1.1  cont.*

A fifth character (as in F31.3; F32.0 and F32.1; F33.0 and F33.1) may be used to specify the presence or absence of the somatic syndrome. To qualify for the somatic syndrome, at least 4 of the following should be present:

- marked loss of interest or pleasure in activities that are normally pleasurable; anhedonia
- lack of emotional reactions to events or activities that normally produce an emotional response
- waking in the morning 2 hours or more before the usual time
- depression worse in the morning
- objective evidence of marked psychomotor retardation or agitation (i.e. remarked on or reported by other people)
- marked loss of appetite
- weight loss (at least 5% of body weight in the past month)
- marked loss of libido

combination of these interventions may be particularly effective in the treatment of depression.[5]

# Decision 1: treatment of choice

Currently available antidepressant medications are all effective for the treatment of depression. Claims that certain agents have a more rapid onset, or are more often associated with remission remain preliminary.[6] Thus, the choice of an antidepressant is often based on tolerability issues and possible side effects. Patients experiencing fewer side effects are more likely to adhere to medication, a crucial consideration given the importance of long-term treatment.

Indeed, newer antidepressants, which show a more favourable side-effect profile than the older tricyclic and tetracyclic agents, are increasingly viewed as the treatment of choice for depression. Among this group, selective serotonin reuptake inhibitors (SSRIs) have been the most extensively studied and used in many countries. Citalopram (20–60 mg/day), escitalopram (10–20 mg/day), fluoxetine (20–40 mg/day), fluvoxamine (100–300 mg/day), paroxetine (20–60 mg/day) and sertraline (50–200 mg/day) all belong to this class of medication.

Recently, antidepressants with a dual mechanism of action affecting both the noradrenergic and serotonergic systems (dual antidepressants) have been introduced, and share, with the SSRIs, a favourable side-effect profile compared with the tricyclic antidepressants. Among this class, venlafaxine (150–300 mg/day) is more a serotonin than a noradrenaline reuptake inhibitor, while milnacipran (50–100 mg/day) is more a noradrenergic than a serotonergic reuptake inhibitor.

Reboxetine (8 mg/day) has been recently introduced as a specific noradrenaline reuptake inhibitor. Mirtazapine (30–60 mg/day) affects both noradrenergic receptors (via $\alpha_2$-blockade) as well as specific serotonergic receptors ($5HT_2$ and $5HT_3$). Nefazodone (200–600 mg/day) affects both 5HT reuptake and the $5HT_2$ receptor (Figure 1.1).

In most countries, tricyclic and tetracyclic antidepressants (e.g. amitriptyline and imipramine) are today considered to be a second-line treatment as they exhibit a burdensome side-effect profile and do not show greater efficacy compared with the newer compounds.[7] The sedating properties of this group of antidepressants, however, still make them a possible choice for clinicians who want to achieve this goal in the acute phase of illness.[8] However, for long-term maintenance pharmacotherapy, better tolerated agents should be prioritized.

Antidepressants are effective for many of the symptom dimensions of depression, and are therefore typically prescribed as monotherapy. Some clinicians would prescribe a short course of benzodiazepines when using a non-sedating antidepressant, particularly when symptoms of anxiety or insomnia are prominent.[9] In patients with psychotic symptoms, addition of an antipsychotic agent is required;[10] presently, the new-generation antipsychotic agents are preferred in view of their favourable side-effect profile.

Antidepressants should be prescribed for an appropriate length of time, and at an appropriate dosage. While there is debate about the length of an adequate trial, some data suggest that a trial of 6–8

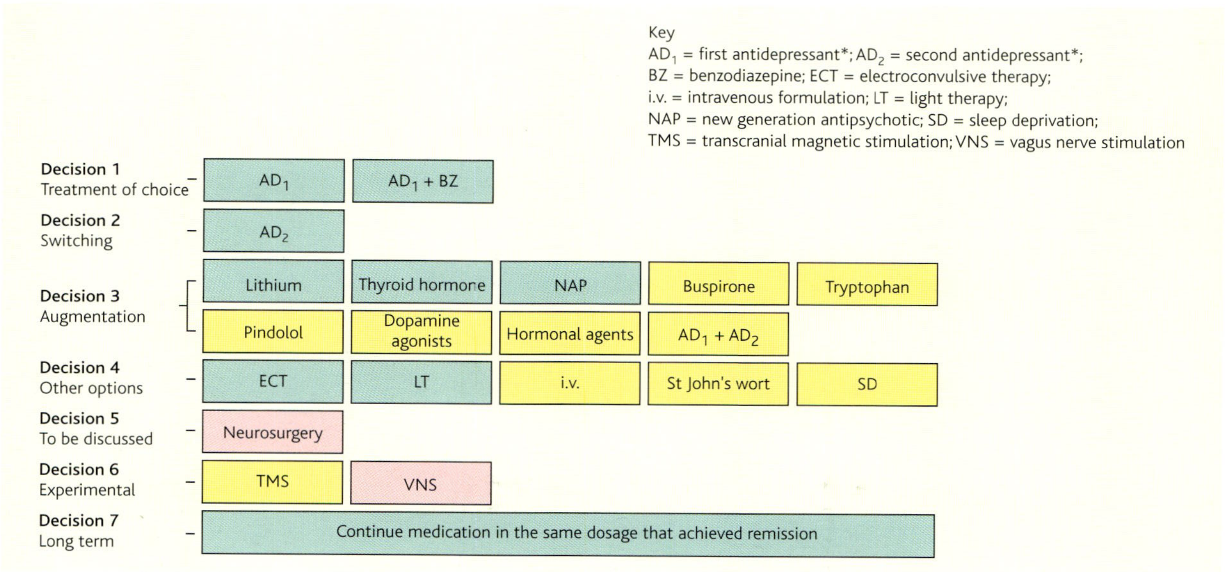

**Figure 1.1** Treatment decisions for unipolar depression. ■ Intervention supported by consistent randomized trials ■ Intervention supported by limited controlled data ■ Intervention supported by uncontrolled data. (*AD₁ denotes treatment of choice; AD₂ suggests using a second AD after a therapeutic attempt with AD₁ has failed.)

5

weeks, or longer, is needed.[11] More severe forms of depression may require higher doses of medication;[12] this is particularly true for many of the older tricyclics, where plasma levels correlate with response. However, even in the case of newer agents, such as the SSRIs, where dose–curve response is comparatively flat, higher doses may be useful in certain patients.

## Decision 2: switching

Should a medication prove ineffective or poorly tolerated, switching to a different medication may be considered. A careful review of baseline symptoms is needed, as side effects are sometimes not easy to differentiate from depressive symptomatology (e.g. dry mouth, headache and nervousness). Once the decision to switch has been made, an antidepressant with different pharmacodynamic properties may be chosen.[13] A number of studies, for example, support the value of switching from one SSRI to a different SSRI. Other strategies, for example, switching from a serotonergic to a noradrenergic agent, seem reasonable and deserve further research.[14]

## Decision 3: augmentation

The question of when to switch and when to augment is one that has received only some empirical study in depression.[15] One approach may, for example, be to switch when there is no response or a partial response to the first trial, to switch or augment if there is a partial response to a second trial, and to augment when there is still no response to a third trial.

The most widely supported augmentation strategies are the addition of lithium and thyroid hormone.[16] There is also growing awareness of the value of certain new generation antipsychotics as augmenting agents in treatment-refractory depression.[17]

A range of other augmenting agents has, however, been studied, including buspirone, tryptophan, pindolol, amphetamines or other dopamine agonists, and oestrogen/testosterone.[18] While uncontrolled augmentation data are often promising, relatively few strategies have been consistently supported by randomized controlled trials.

One theoretical approach to augmentation is to use an antidepressant that has a different mechanism of action from the first medication.[19] For example, there is some support for adding an agent with a noradrenergic mechanism of action (e.g. reboxetine) to an SSRI, or for combining a RIMA with an SSRI.[18]

Combinations of medication may also be used, not so much to augment antidepressant response, but to target particular depressive symptoms, based on the therapeutic profile of the added agent. For example, if loss of sleep is reported, trazodone or mianserin, which have sedative effects, can be added.

Further empirical data are, however, needed to support these theoretical approaches. Furthermore, interactions via the cytochrome P450 system or enzyme-induction (such as with carbamazepine) need to be considered. The combination of irreversible MAOIs with SSRIs, in particular, is contraindicated due to possible side effects.

## Decision 4: other options

For delusional depression and treatment-refractory depression, electroconvulsive therapy (ECT) may be highly effective.[20] ECT is also helpful in moderate-to-severe depression.

Light therapy (e.g. 10,000 lux for 0.5–1 h/day or 2500 lux for 2–4 h/day) is the treatment of choice for seasonal affective disorder and, in combination with pharmacotherapy, a possible additive treatment strategy for non-seasonal depression.[21]

Some psychiatrists in Europe have a preference for intravenous antidepressants, a practice that is not, however, endorsed by most Anglo-American clinicians and researchers. Support for intravenous formulations is based in part on placebo-controlled studies suggesting that these have a faster onset of action.

A few preparations of St John's wort in high concentration (e.g. Jarsin or Neuroplant 900 mg/day) have been demonstrated in randomized controlled trials to be effective in mild-to-moderate depression.[22]

Sleep deprivation (SD) has been studied in controlled trials in research settings, and appears to be effective in the treatment of depression.

## Decision 5: treatments to be discussed

Specific stereotactic techniques might prove to be helpful in the neurosurgical treatment of severe forms of treatment-refractory depression.

## Decision 6: experimental approaches

Transcranial magnetic stimulation (TMS) has been studied for its possible clinical applicability. Although statistically significant treatment effects have been found in open and controlled trials, a clinically meaningful response has not yet been demonstrated. Technically, repeated rhythmic TMS (repetitive or rTMS) seems to be the most effective technique. Further studies are necessary to clarify the relevant methodology and the regions of the brain that should be stimulated.

Some authors believe that vagus nerve stimulation (VNS) may ultimately prove useful, but this has to be proven in positive randomized controlled trials.

## Decision 7: long-term approach

Antidepressant medication used in the acute phase should be continued in the same dosage for at least 6–9 months after the onset of a clinical response (*continuation phase*), in order to prevent the re-emergence or relapse of the index episode of major depression. In addition, many patients may require further treatment, at this same dose, in order to prevent recurrence of further episodes of major depression (*maintenance* or *prophylactic phase*).[23]

Given that depression is a chronic illness, national and international consensus conferences have increasingly emphasized the importance of maintenance therapy, particularly in patients with prior or severe episodes. One rule, for example, would be that depressed patients with either three episodes (including the index episode) or two episodes (where one was very severe with, for instance, a high degree of suicidality or genetic predisposition) should receive long-term treatment for at least 5 years.[24] Given the difficulty of conducting long-term randomized controlled trials, such rules reflect clinical consensus rather than the results of studies specifically designed to address the length of treatment.

The favourable side-effect profile of newer antidepressants promotes adherence to therapeutic doses of the medication. As discussed earlier, newer medications therefore have an advantage over the older tri- and tetracyclic antidepressants in maintenance therapy.[25]

Psychotherapy may play a useful role during maintenance pharmacotherapy. Nevertheless, there is a relative paucity of studies examining the optimal combination and sequencing of pharmacotherapy and psychotherapy over the long term.

# References

1. Kasper S, Möller HJ, Müller-Spahn F. *Depression. Diagnose und Pharmakotherapie*. Stuttgart: Thieme-Verlag, 1997.
2. Kessler RC, McGonagle KC, Zhao S, et al. Lifetime and 12-month prevalence of DSM-III-R psychiatric disorders in the United States: results from the National Comorbidity Survey. *Arch Gen Psychiatry* 1994; **51**:8–19.
3. Kasper S, (ed.). European algorithm project. *Int J Psychiatry Clin Pract* 1997; **1**(1):S1–S30.
4. Brunello N, Burrows G, Jönsson B, et al. Critical issues in the treatment of affective disorders. *Depression* 1995; **3**:187–98.
5. Keller MB, McCullough JP, Klein DN, et al. A comparison of nefazodone, cognitive behavioral analysis system of psychotherapy, and their combination for the treatment of chronic depression. *N Eng J Med* 2000; **342**:1462–70.
6. Gelenberg AJ, Chesen CL. How fast are antidepressants. *J Clin Psychiatry* 2000; **61**:712–21.
7. Kasper S, Lépine JP, Mendlewicz J, et al. Efficacy, safety and indications for tricyclic and newer antidepressants. *Depression* 1994/5;

2:127–37.

8. Chan CH, Janicak PG, Davis JM. Response of psychotic and non-psychotic depressed patients to tricyclic antidepressants. *J Clin Psychiatry* 1987; **48**:197–200.

9. Furukawa TA, Streiner DL, Young LT. Antidepressant plus benzodiazepine for major depression (Cochrane Review). *Cochrane Database Syst Rev* 2001; **2**:CD001026.

10. Rothschild AJ, Samson JA, Bessette MP, et al. Efficacy of the combination of fluoxetine and perphenazine in the treatment of psychotic depression. *J Clin Psychiatry* 1993; **54**:338–42.

11. Donovan SJ, Quitkin FM, Stewart JW, et al. Duration of antidepressant trials: clinical and research implications. *J Clin Psychopharmacol* 1994; **14**:64–6.

12. Paykel ES, Hollyman JA, Freeling P, et al. Predictors of therapeutic benefit from amitriptyline in mild depression: a general practice placebo-controlled trial. *J Affect Disorder* 1988; **14**:83–5.

13. Thase ME, Rush J, Howland RH, et al. Double-blind switch study of imipramine or sertraline treatment of antidepressant-resistant chronic depression. *Arch Gen Psychiatry* 2002; **59**:233–9

14. Marangell LB. Switching antidepressants for treatment-resistant major depression. *J Clin Psychiatry* 2001; **62**(Suppl.18):12–17.

15. Nelson JC. Treatment of antidepressant nonresponders: augmentation or switch. *J Clin Psychiatry* 1998; **59**(Suppl.):35–41.

16. Joffe RT, Singer W, Levitt AJ, et al. A placebo-controlled trial comparison of lithium and triiodothyronine augmentation of tricyclic antidepressants in unipolar refractory depression. *Arch Gen Psychiatry* 1993; **50**:387–93.

17. Tohen M, Shelton R, Tollefson GD, et al. Olanzapine plus fluoxetine: double-blind and open-label results in treatment-resistant major depressive disorder. *European Neuropsychopharmacol* 1999; **9**(Suppl.5):S246.

18. Fava M. Augmentation and combination strategies in treatment-resistant depression. *J Clin Psychiatry* 2001; **62**(Suppl.18):4–11.

19. Nelson JC. Augmentation strategies with serotonergic-noradrenergic combinations. *J Clin Psychiatry* 1998; **59**(Suppl.):65–8.

20. Abrams R. *Electroconvulsive Therapy*. 2nd edn. New York, Oxford: Oxford University Press, 1992.

21. Kasper S, Neumeister A. Non-pharmacological treatments for depression: focus on sleep deprivation and light therapy. In: Briley M, Montgomery S, eds. *Antidepressant Therapy: At the dawn of the third millennium*. London: Martin Dunitz, 1998:255–78.

22. LaFrance WC, Lauterbach EC, Coffey EC, et al. The use of herbal alternative medicines in neuropsychiatry. *J Neuropsychiatr Clin Neurosci* 2000; **12**:177–92.

23. Frank E, Kupfer DJ, Perel JM, et al. Maintenance therapies on recurrent depression protocol: treatment outcome. *Arch Gen Psychiatry* 1990; **47**: 1093–9.

24. Kasper S. The rationale for long-term antidepressant therapy. *Int Clin Psychopharmacol* 1993; **8**:225–35.

25. Montgomery SA. Selective serotonin re-uptake inhibitors in long-term treatment of depression. In: Feighner JP and Boyer WF, eds. *Perspectives in Psychiatry*. vol.5 *Selective Serotonin Re-Uptake Inhibitors*. 2nd edn. Chichester: Wiley, 1996:123–33.

# Pharmacotherapy of bipolar disorder

## Introduction

Bipolar disorder is a severe and chronic psychiatric disorder.[1–3] Patients may experience substantial distress and impairment, and are at risk for significant morbidity and mortality (after suicide).[4] Most patients require some level of long-term psychiatric care.[5,6] The diagnoses of bipolar I (i.e. the criteria for major depression and mania are met), as well as bipolar II (i.e. the criteria for major depression and hypomania are met), are described in DSM-IV. The criteria for major depression/depressive episode are shown in Table 1.1 (on page 2) and those for mania in Table 2.1.

Epidemiological studies have substantiated that the lifetime prevalence rate of bipolar disorder is between 1 and 5% (1% is the lower limit and 5% allows inclusion of a bipolar spectrum).[7] The diagnosis of bipolar spectrum disorders (not meeting the threshold for bipolar I disorder) is of clinical relevance since these conditions may also respond to treatment with mood stabilizers.[5,8] A hypomanic episode secondary to antidepressant treatment, for example, does not indicate a diagnosis of bipolar disorder in DSM-IV, but does suggest that a bipolar course has been uncovered by an antidepressant treatment.

Clinical decisions pertaining to the treatment of bipolar disorder can be grouped around the topics of:

- depression
- mania
- rapid cycling/mixed states (Table 2.1).

*Table 2.1* *Diagnostic criteria for mania.*

| DSM-IV criteria for a single manic episode |
|---|

**Note** This is part of the bipolar I disorder (code 296.0x)

A. Abnormal and persistently elevated, expansive, or irritable mood, lasting at least 1 week

B. Episode includes three (or more) of the following symptoms (four if the mood is only irritable) that have been present to a significant degree:
- inflated self-esteem or grandiosity
- decreased need for sleep (e.g. feels rested after only 3 hours' sleep)
- more talkative
- racing thoughts
- distractibility
- increase in goal-directed activity or psychomotor agitation
- over-involvement in pleasurable activities that have a high risk of painful consequences (e.g. unrestrained buying sprees, sexual indiscretions, or foolish business investments)

C. Symptoms do not meet criteria for a mixed episode

D. Episode sufficiently severe to markedly impair work and social activities or to necessitate hospitalization, or psychotic features present

E. Symptoms are not caused by a substance (e.g. drug or hormone)

| ICD-10 criteria for mania (category F30) |
|---|

A. Mood must be predominantly elevated, expansive or irritable, and definitely abnormal for the individual concerned. The mood change must be prominent and sustained for at least 1 week (unless it is severe enough to require hospitalization)

B. At least three of the following must be present (four if the mood is merely irritable), leading to severe interference with personal functioning in daily living:
- increased activity or physical restlessness
- increased talkativeness ('pressure of speech')
- flight of ideas or the subjective experience of thoughts racing
- loss of normal social inhibitions, resulting in behaviour inappropriate to circumstances
- reduced need for sleep
- inflated self-esteem or grandiosity

*Table 2.1 cont.*

- distractibility or constant changes in activity or plans
- foolish or reckless behaviour where the individual does not recognize the risks, e.g. spending sprees, foolish enterprises, reckless driving
- marked sexual energy or sexual indiscretion

C. There are no hallucinations or delusions, although perceptual disorders may occur (e.g. subjective hyperacusis), appreciation of colours as especially vivid

D. Most commonly used exclusion clause: the episode is not attributable to psychoactive substance abuse (categories F10–F19) or to any organic mental disorder (F00–F09)

*Table 2.2 Mood stabilizers for prophylactic treatment in bipolar disorder.*

| Agent | Dosage (mg/day)* | Serum level |
|---|---|---|
| Lithium | 400–800 | 0.6–0.8 mmol/l |
| Carbamazepine | 400–1200 | 17—42 µmol/l (4–10 µg/ml) |
| Valproic acid | 750–1500 | 50–120 µg/ml |
| Sodium valproate | | 350–700 µmol/l |
| Lamotrigine** | 200–400 | 1–10 µg/ml |

\* Initial dose may be substantially lower
\*\* Not yet licensed for this indication

# Decision 1: treatment of choice

## Depression

Lithium (up to 1 mmol/l) appears effective in the treatment of bipolar depression.[8] Furthermore, certain other mood stabilizers, such as lamotrigine, may also be effective here.[9] Many clinicians would only consider the addition of an antidepressant once treatment with a mood stabilizer is already under way. In choosing an antidepressant, evidence that the SSRIs and other newer agents are associated with a lower switch rate to mania than the older tricyclics should be taken into account.

## Mania

Mood stabilizers are effective in the treatment of manic episodes. While lithium (up to 1 mmol/l) and valproic acid (50–120 µg/ml) have long been shown useful,[8,9] there is increasing evidence that other agents (e.g. carbamazepine, lamotrigine) may also be effective.[9]

Antipsychotic medications and benzodiazepines (e.g. clonazepam) are often used in combination with mood stabilizers. New generation antipsychotics are preferred in view of their superior tolerability profile, and indeed some of these agents have been shown effective for the treatment of manic episodes in randomized controlled trials.[10]

## Rapid cycling/mixed episodes

If rapid cycling occurs (e.g. at least four episodes of depression or mania a year),[11] or mixed episodes occur (Table 2.1), the use of mood stabilizers rather than antidepressants is recommended.[12] Furthermore, valproate may be more effective for rapid cycling/mixed episodes than lithium. A new generation antipsychotic is also often added.[13]

# Decision 2: switching

## Depression

When the combination of a mood stabilizer and an antidepressant proves ineffective or poorly tolerated in bipolar depression, switching to a different regime may be considered – for example, switching the antidepressant to another with a different mechanism of action.[14] Thus, if SSRIs are the first choice, a noradrenergic or specific serotonergic/noradrenergic (dual- or specific-acting) antidepressant could be chosen.[15] There are, however, few controlled trials which study the value of such strategies, and augmentation is often favoured in clinical practice. Diagnostic re-evaluation is also necessary in order to prevent misdiagnosis.[16]

## Mania

When the combination of a mood stabilizer and an antipsychotic/benzodiazepine proves ineffective or poorly tolerated in mania, switching to a different regime may be considered. For example, in patients with extra-pyramidal symptoms (EPS) secondary to older antipsychotic agents, switching to a new generation antipsychotic may be advisable. Again, there are few studies that rigorously compare different strategies, such as switching mood stabilizers, in this situation, and augmentation is often favoured in clinical practice.[17]

# Decision 3: augmentation

## Depression

When the combination of a mood stabilizer and an antidepressant proves ineffective in bipolar depression, augmentation with a second mood stabilizer or other agent may be considered.[18] Thyroid hormone, for example, has been used in this context.[19] There is, however, a paucity of controlled trials on augmentation strategies in bipolar depression.

## Mania

When the combination of a mood stabilizer and an antipsychotic/benzodiazepine proves ineffective in bipolar mania, augmentation with a second mood stabilizer may be considered. Although there are, again, relatively few controlled studies of such strategies, polypharmacy for the treatment of mania is not uncommon in clinical practice.

## Rapid cycling

In rapid-cycling bipolar disorder,[13] when the combination of a mood stabilizer and an antipsychotic proves ineffective, the addition of a second mood stabilizer may be merited (e.g. the combination of valproate and carbamazepine). In some cases, use of three mood stabilizers needs to be considered (e.g. lithium, carbamazepine and valproic acid), although caution about drug interactions is required. The addition of thyroid hormone may also be useful in such cases.[20,21]

# Decision 4: other options

## Depression

ECT is an effective treatment for severe depression in general and also for bipolar depression. If symptoms are very severe, with retardation and psychotic features, ECT may be regarded as a first-line treatment.

Although there are few empirical data, some clinicians favour the use of intravenous antidepressants for bipolar depression.

## Mania

ECT is also effective in the treatment of mania.[22]

# Decision 5: treatments to be discussed

Nimodipine[23] and verapamil[24] are other options if major depression is frequently accompanied by manic phases. Nevertheless, the data available are currently inconsistent.

# Decision 6: experimental approaches

Transcranial magnetic stimulation (TMS) is currently under investigation as a treatment for bipolar depression. The practical applicability for everyday clinical practice, however, has not been established.

Not all anticonvulsants have been adequately studied in bipolar disorder. Further work with topiramate, gabapentin, tiagabin and other newer agents is needed.[9]

# Decision 7: long-term approach

If, after a *depressive phase*, euthymia has been achieved with a mood stabilizer together with antidepressant treatment, the mood stabilizer (either one or several) should be continued. Although many US authors favour the cessation of antidepressants as soon as euthymia has been reached, some European psychiatrists tend to continue antidepressant medication for a somewhat longer period. Additional data are needed to determine the optimal strategy.[25]

If euthymia has been achieved after a *manic state* of the illness, older antipsychotic medications (e.g. haloperidol) should be discontinued in order to prevent depression. However, it might be suggested that the new generation antipsychotic agents can be continued for a longer period of time as they may have antidepressant effects.

If euthymia has been achieved in *rapid cycling*, the same treatment regimen should be continued, and antidepressant agents should be avoided.

Psychotherapy may play an important role in the long-term treatment of bipolar disorder. The aims of this intervention include: establishing and maintaining a therapeutic alliance; providing information on bipolar illness; monitoring the patient's psychiatric status; recommending regular patterns of activity and wakefulness; identifying psychosocial stressors and helping adaptation to them; early identification of new episodes; and inclusion of the patient's family or other social support.

Long-term pharmacotherapy with mood stabilizers alone is indicated for most cases of bipolar I disorder. For bipolar II disorder, one rule may be to continue prophylactic treatment if three episodes of depression or hypomania have occurred on a lifetime basis, or if two episodes of depression or hypomania have occurred within the previous 5 years (Figures 2.1 and 2.2).

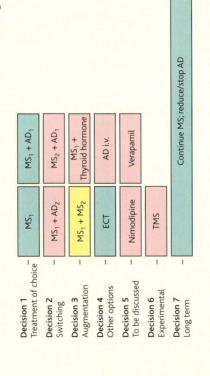

**Figure 2.1** *Treatment decisions for bipolar depression.* ■ *Intervention supported by consistent randomized trials* ■ *Intervention supported by limited controlled data* ■ *Intervention supported by uncontrolled data.* ■ *Intervention supported by uncontrolled data.* (*$MS_1/AD_1$ denotes treatment of choice; $MS_2/AD_2$ suggests using a second MS/AD after a therapeutic attempt with $MS_1/AD_1$ has failed.*)

Key
$AD_1$ = first antidepressant*; $AD_2$ = second antidepressant*;
ECT = electroconvulsive therapy; i.v. = intravenous formulation;
$MS_1$ = first mood stabilizer*; $MS_2$ = second mood stabilizer*;
TMS = transcranial magnetic stimulation

**Decision 1**
Treatment of choice – | $MS_1$ | $MS_1 + AD_1$

**Decision 2**
Switching – | $MS_1 + AD_2$ | $MS_2 + AD_1$

**Decision 3**
Augmentation – | $MS_1 + MS_2$ | $MS_1 +$ Thyroid hormone

**Decision 4**
Other options – | ECT | AD i.v.

**Decision 5**
To be discussed – | Nimodipine | Verapamil

**Decision 6**
Experimental – | TMS

**Decision 7**
Long term – | Continue MS; reduce/stop AD

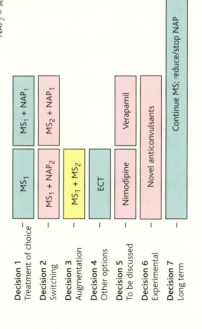

Key

AD = antidepressant; ECT = electroconvulsive therapy;
$MS_1$ = first mood stabilizer*; $MS_2$ = first mood stabilizer*;
$NAP_1$ = first new generation antipsychotic*;
$NAP_2$ = second new generation antipsychotic*

| Decision 1 Treatment of choice | – | $MS_1$ | $MS_1 + NAP_1$ |
| Decision 2 Switching | – | $MS_1 + NAP_2$ | $MS_2 + NAP_1$ |
| Decision 3 Augmentation | – | $MS_1 + MS_2$ | |
| Decision 4 Other options | – | ECT | |
| Decision 5 To be discussed | – | Nimodipine | Verapamil |
| Decision 6 Experimental | – | Novel anticonvulsants | |
| Decision 7 Long term | – | Continue MS; reduce/stop NAP | |

Intervention supported by consistent randomized trials ■  Intervention supported by limited controlled data ■  Intervention supported by uncontrolled data. ■

*Figure 2.2* Treatment decisions for mania. ■ Intervention supported by consistent randomized trials ■ Intervention supported by limited controlled data ■ Intervention supported by uncontrolled data. (*$MS_1$/$NAP_1$ denotes treatment of choice; $MS_2$/$NAP_2$ suggests using a second MS/NAP after a therapeutic attempt with $MS_1$/$NAP_1$ has failed.)

# References

1. Goodwin FK, Jamison KR. *Manic-depressive illness*. New York: Oxford University Press, 1990.

2. Angst J, Marneros A. Bipolarity from ancient to modern times: conception, birth, and rebirth. *J Affect Disord* 2001; **67**:3–19

3. Weckerly J. Pediatric bipolar mood disorder. *J Dev Behav Pediatr* 2002; **23**:42–56.

4. Angst J, Sellaro Rd, Angst F. Long-term outcome and mortality of treated versus untreated bipolar and depressed patients: a preliminary report. *Int J Psychiatry Clin Pract* 1998; **2**:115–19.

5. Kasper S, Haushofer M, Zapotoczky HG, et al. Konsensus-Statement: Diagnostik und Therapie der bipolaren Störung. *Neuropsychiatrie* 1999; **13**:100–8.

6. Müller-Oerlinghausen B, Ahrens B, Grof E, et al. The effect of long-term lithium treatment on the mortality of patients with manic-depressive and schizoaffective illness. *Acta Psychiatr Scand* 1992; **86**:218–22.

7. Kessler RC, McGonagle KC, Zhao S, et al. Lifetime and 12-month prevalence of DSM-III-R psychiatric disorders in the United States: results from the National Comorbidity Survey. *Arch Gen Psychiatry* 1994; **51**:8–19.

8. Schou M. *Lithium Treatment of Manic-Depressive Illness: A practical guide*. 5th edn. New York: S. Karger, 1993.

9. Calabrese JR, Shelton MD, Rapport DJ, et al. Bipolar disorders and the effectiveness of novel anticonvulsants. *J Clin Psychiatry* 2002; **63**(Suppl.3):5–9.

10. Yatham LN. The role of novel antipsychotics in bipolar disorders. *J Clin Psychiatry* 2002; **63**(Suppl.3):10–14.

11. Maj M, Magliano L, Pirozzi R, et al. Validity of rapid cycling as a course specifier for bipolar disorder. *Am J Psychiatry* 1994; **151**:1015–19.

12. Wehr TA, Goodwin FK. Can antidepressants cause mania and worsen the course of affective illness? *Am J Psychiatry* 1987; **144**:1403–11.

13. Calabrese JR, Woyshville MJ. A medication algorithm for treatment of bipolar rapid cycling. *J Clin Psychiatry* 1995; **56**:11–18.

14. Cole AJ, Scott J, Ferrier IN, Eccleston D. Patterns of treatment resistance in bipolar affective disorder. *Acta Psychiatr Scand* 1993; **88**:121–3.

15. Goodwin GM, Bourgeois ML, Conti L, et al. Treatment of bipolar depressive mood disorders: algorithms for pharmacotherapy. *Int J Psychiatry Clin Pract* 1997; **1**:S9–S12.

16. Post RM, Roy-Byrne PP, Uhde TW. Graphic representation of the life course of illness in patients with affective disorder. *Am J Psychiatry* 1988; **145**:844–8.

17. Walden J, Heßlinger B. Bedeutung alter und neuer Antiepileptika in der Behandlung psychischere Erkrankungen. *Fortschr Neurol Psychiat* 1995; **63**:320–35.

18. Keck PE Jr, McElroy SL, Vuckovic A, et al. Combined valproate and carbamazepine treatment of bipolar disorder. *J Neuropsychiatry Clin Neurosci* 1992; **4**:319–22.

19. Baumgartner A, Bauer M, Hellweg R. Treatment of intractable non-rapid cycling bipolar affective disorder with high-dose thyroxine: an open clinical trial. *Neuropsychopharmacol* 1994; **10**:183–9.

20. Baumgartner A. Thyroxine and the treatment of affective disorders: an overview of the results of basic and clinical research. *Int J Neuropsychopharm* 2000; **3**:149–65.

21. Calabrese JR, Shelton MD, Rapport DJ, et al. Current research on rapid cycling bipolar disorder and its treatment. *J Affect Disord* 2001; **67**:241–55.

22. American Psychiatric Association. *The Practice of Electroconvulsive Therapy: Recommendations for treatment, training and privileging: a task force report of the American Psychiatric Association*. Washington DC: American Psychiatric Press, 1990.

23. Pazzaglia PJ, Post RM, Ketter TA, et al. Preliminary controlled trial of nimodipine in ultra-rapid cycling affective dysregulation. *Psychiatry Res* 1993; **49**:257–72.

24. Höschl C, Kozeny J. Verapamil in affective disorders: a controlled, double-blind study. *Biol Psychiatry* 1989; **25**:128–40.

25. Altshuler L, Kiriakos L, Calcagno J, et al. The impact of antidepressant discontinuation versus antidepression continuation on 1-year risk for relapse of bipolar depression: a retrospective chart review. *J Clin Psychiatry* 2001; **62**:612–16.

# Pharmacotherapy of schizophrenia

3

## Introduction

Schizophrenia represents a clinically heterogeneous nosological entity which is responsive to medication in the short and long term.[1–3] The positive and negative symptoms of schizophrenia have long been described, with more recent literature emphasizing also depressive and cognitive symptom dimensions.[4] Epidemiological studies from around the world have indicated that schizophrenia affects approximately 1% of the general population, regardless of race and developmental status of the individual country (Table 3.1).

Since the 1950s, several neuroleptic (antipsychotic) drugs of high and low potency have been available for acute and long-term (maintenance) therapy. Randomized controlled trials have shown the superiority of these medications compared with placebo. The introduction of a new generation of antipsychotic agents (amisulpride, clozapine, olanzapine, risperidone, quetiapine, sertindole, ziprasidone, zotepine) has led to further progress towards the successful treatment of schizophrenia.

The defining characteristics of these so-called 'atypical antipsychotics' remain controversial. Early theories posited that both dopamine-blocking and serotonin antagonist activities were important, while more recent work has suggested that some of these agents have rapid dissociation from dopamine receptors. From a practical perspective, however, there is growing evidence that many of the new generation agents are not only more effective for negative, cognitive and depressive symptoms, but are also associated with fewer or even no extrapyramidal symptoms (EPS).[5,6] They therefore represent a key advance.

*Table 3.1* *Diagnostic criteria for schizophrenia.*

| DMS-IV criteria for schizophrenia (code 295.xx) |
| --- |
| A. Characteristic symptoms: two* (or more) of the following, each present for a significant portion of time during 1 month (or less if treated successfully):<br>• delusions<br>• hallucinations<br>• disorganized speech (e.g. frequent derailment or incoherence)<br>• grossly disorganized or catatonic behaviour<br>• negative symptoms (affective flattening, alogia, or avolition)<br><br>* If delusions are bizarre or hallucinations consist of a voice keeping up a running commentary on the person's behaviour or thoughts, or two or more voices conversing with each other, only one symptom is needed for a diagnosis |
| B. Social/occupational dysfunction in work, interpersonal relations, or self-care most of the time |
| C. Duration: continuous signs of the disturbance persist for at least 6 months: **must** include at least 1 month of symptoms (or less if treated successfully) that meet criterion active-phase symptoms and **may** include periods of prodromal or residual symptoms during which only negative symptoms or two or more symptoms in an attenuated form (e.g. odd beliefs, unusual perceptual experiences) may be present |
| D. Exclude schizoaffective disorder and mood disorder with psychotic features because either:<br>• no major depressive, manic, or mixed episodes have occurred concurrently with active-phase symptoms; or<br>• if, during active-phase, symptoms are brief relative to length of active and residual periods |
| E. Exclude effects caused by a substance (e.g. drug or hormone) or general medical condition |
| F. If history of autistic disorder or other pervasive developmental disorder, the additional diagnosis of schizophrenia is made only if prominent delusions or hallucinations are also present for at least 1 month (or less if treated successfully) |

*Table 3.1* cont.

### ICD-10 criteria for schizophrenia (category F20.0–F20.3)

General criteria for paranoid, hebephrenic, catatonic, and undifferentiated schizophrenia

A.  At least one of the syndromes, symptoms, and signs listed under (1), or at least two of the symptoms and signs listed under (2) should be present for most of the time during an episode of psychotic illness lasting for at least 1 month (or at some time during most of the days)

(1)  At least one of the following must be present:
- thought echo, thought insertion or withdrawal, or thought broadcasting
- delusions of control, influence or passivity, clearly referred to body or limb movements or specific thoughts, actions or sensations; delusional perception
- hallucinatory voices giving a running commentary on the patient's behaviour, or discussing the patient between themselves, or other types of hallucinatory voices coming from some part of the body
- persistent delusions of other kinds that are culturally inappropriate and completely impossible, e.g. being able to control the weather, being in communication with aliens

(2)  Or at least two of the following:
- persistent hallucinations in any modality, when occurring everyday for at least 1 month, when accompanied by delusions (which may be fleeting or half formed) without clear affective content, or when accompanied by persistent overvalued ideas
- neologisms, breaks or interpolations in the train of thought, resulting in incoherence or irrelevant speech
- catatonic behaviour, such as excitement, posturing or waxy flexibility, negativism, mutism and stupor
- 'negative' symptoms, such as marked apathy, paucity of speech and blunting or incongruity of emotional responses (it must be clear that these are not due to depression or to neuroleptic medication)

*cont.*

*Table 3.1 cont.*

B.   Most commonly used exclusion clauses:
  •   if the patient also meets the criteria for manic episode (category F30.x) or depressive episode (F32.x), the criteria listed under (1) and (2) above must have been met before the disturbance of mood developed
  •   the disorder is not attributable to organic brain disease (in the sense of F00–F09) or to alcohol- or drug-related intoxication (F1x.0), dependence (F1x.2) or withdrawal (F1x.3 and F1x.4)

# Decision 1: treatment of choice

Given the growing literature indicating that the new generation antipsychotics are effective for a broader range of symptoms (positive as well as negative, depressive and cognitive symptoms) and have fewer EPS than older agents, these 'atypical antipsychotics' can be considered the pharmacotherapy of choice in schizophrenia. The traditional agents may have a role in settings where they are the only affordable agents, or in particular patients where they have demonstrated clear efficacy and tolerability.

The new-generation antipsychotics have rather different pharmacological properties, with varying effects at a range of different neurotransmitter receptors. While the number of studies comparing different new generation antipsychotics remains limited, from a clinical perspective it is worth considering potential differences when choosing an agent. Thus, for example, in an agitated patient, a more sedating agent may be useful. (In clinical practice, adjunctive benzodiazepines are also often used during the acute phase of treatment.) Similarly, in patients with weight problems, an agent with less associated weight gain may be tried first.

Antipsychotic trials should be of adequate dose and duration. In first-episode patients, there is evidence that lower doses than usual may be effective. Indeed, there is a growing emphasis on providing treatment for longer periods rather than using very high doses (as was once common); trials should be at least 4–6 weeks long, although there is some evidence that symptoms continue to improve for several months after initiation of certain antipsychotic agents. Individual patients may, however, require relatively higher doses before responding.

## Decision 2: switching

Should a particular antipsychotic prove ineffective (e.g. <20% improvement on standard rating scales), or poorly tolerated, a different agent should be considered. Factors that may be associated with a lack of response (e.g. comorbid disorders, psychosocial stressors, non-adherence) should of course be reviewed. There is, however, a growing literature supporting the value of switching from a traditional agent to a new-generation antipsychotic agent. There are persuasive data, for example, that clozapine is effective in patients who have failed to respond to different traditional antipsychotics.[7] There is also a growing database suggesting the efficacy of certain other new generation agents in patients resistant to treatment with older antipsychotics,[8] and there is evidence that switching from a typical agent to a new generation medication can be accompanied by improved toleration of medication.[9]

While the literature on switching between the various new-generation antipsychotic agents is less well developed, the different pharmacological and side-effect profiles of these medications provide a clinical rationale for also switching between these agents in relevant patients. Again, for example, it may be possible to decrease sedation, or reduce weight gain, by switching between the new generation agents. Such considerations may become particularly important during long-term treatment.

## Decision 3: augmentation

The question of when to switch and when to augment is one that remains understudied. Work showing that patients who are resistant to traditional antipsychotics may respond to new-generation antipsychotic agents in general, and to clozapine in particular, supports the initial use of a switching strategy in treatment-resistant schizophrenia. However, there is also a range of randomized controlled augmentation studies, suggesting that that approach may also be useful in some cases.

When augmentation is effective, a range of symptom dimensions may improve. Nevertheless, there is a clinical rationale for attempting to target particular symptoms with relevant augmentation approaches. Thus, for example, augmentation of an antipsychotic with a benzodiazepine may be useful in patients with anxiety symptoms or sleeping problems.[10] Similarly, lithium and anticonvulsants (carbamazepine or valproate) may be useful in augmenting typical antipsychotics in patients with aggressive/agitated symptoms or with schizoaffective disorder.[11] There is also some interest in adding low doses of high-potency traditional antipsychotics to new generation agents to improve efficacy, although this strategy has not been well studied to date.

In patients with schizophrenia and comorbid disorders, the use of relevant combinations of different medications can be considered. For example, addition of antidepressants to antipsychotics may be useful in 'post-psychotic' depression.[12] Similarly, in schizophrenia with obsessive-compulsive disorder, addition of selective serotonin reuptake inhibitors (SSRIs) to antipsychotic medication may be effective.

Further research is needed to clarify the relative value of different augmentation strategies in the treatment of schizophrenia without comorbidity. Furthermore, it is important to be aware of potential drug–drug interactions when using polypharmacy.[13] The addition of fluvoxamine to clozapine, for example, may result in higher serum levels of clozapine, as both agents are metabolized by the P450 system. The combination of antipsychotics with antidepressants may also result in an increase in hallucinations and conceptual disorganization.[14]

Some authorities believe that buspirone augmentation is useful, but again controlled studies are required.

## Decision 4: other options

Depot formulations with a relatively short (e.g. 2–3 days with zuclopenthixol) or longer (e.g. 2–4 weeks with fluphenazine decanoate and haloperidol decanoate) duration have a role in some patients. In severe, uncooperative patients, parenteral administration may play a crucial role in promoting adherence to treatment. This strategy can perhaps also be applied if there is a poor response to an oral antipsychotic due to poor absorption and/or rapid first-pass metabolism, although this has not been systematically studied to date.

## Decision 5: treatments to be discussed

Electroconvulsive therapy (ECT) is effective in patients with catatonia, severe excitement, psychotic aggression, or extremely disturbing symptoms that do not respond to medication. For patients without such psychopathology, ECT is not indicated.

## Decision 6: experimental approaches

Psychotropics with specific mechanisms of action are presently being intensively investigated to provide a more effective treatment for differing dimensions of schizophrenia (positive, negative, depressive and cognitive symptoms), together with a favourable side-effect profile. These mechanisms include σ-receptor antagonists and $5HT_2$ antagonists, which offer the potential of reducing dopamine synthesis and blocking cortical $5HT_2$, as well as glutamate agonists, cannabis antagonists and neuroreceptor-modulating agents. The 'atypical antipsychotics' have moved the field beyond a simplistic dopamine theory of schizophrenia, and such newer agents may lead to correspondingly novel understandings of this disorder.

## Decision 7: long-term approach

Long-term studies of traditional agents have been available for some time, and there is now a growing database on the long-term use of new-generation antipsychotic agents. On the one hand, reduction of dosage or intermittent treatment is associated with an increased rate of relapse.[15] On the other hand, in clinically stable

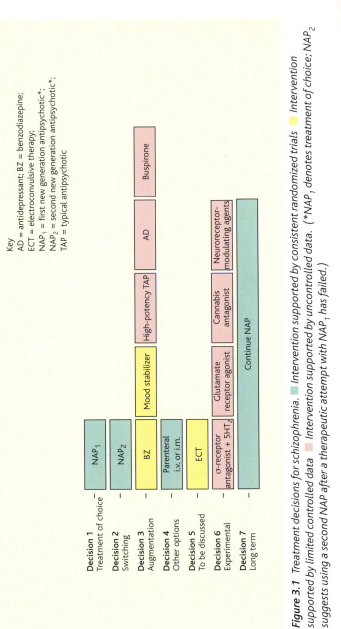

**Figure 3.1** *Treatment decisions for schizophrenia.* ■ *Intervention supported by consistent randomized trials.* ■ *Intervention supported by limited controlled data.* ■ *Intervention supported by uncontrolled data.* (*$NAP_1$ denotes treatment of choice; $NAP_2$ suggests using a second NAP after a therapeutic attempt with $NAP_1$ has failed.*)

patients a gradual tapering of medication to determine a minimally effective dose may be advised.[16] Treatment can be divided into an acute phase lasting 6–8 weeks, followed by a stabilization (continuation treatment) phase of at least 6 months in which the patient exhibits a high degree of psychobiological vulnerability, and finally by a maintenance phase (prophylactic treatment) continuing for 2 years or longer. In many cases a life-long treatment with specific psychiatric management tailored to the individual needs of the patient is necessary.[16] Specific psychotherapy, focusing on the cognitive and psychosocial impairment of the patient, together with an optimal pharmacotherapy, maximizes the long-term outcome (Figure 3.1).

# References

1. American Psychiatric Association. Practice guidelines for the treatment of patients with schizophrenia. *Am J Psychiatry* 1997; **154**(Suppl.4):1–63.
2. Altamura AC, Barnas C, Bitter I, et al. Treatment of schizophrenic disorders; algorithms for acute pharmacotherapy. *Int J Psychiatr Clin Pract* 1997; **1**:S25–S30.
3. Kasper S. *Sicher Therapieren mit Neuroleptika. 3. Ausgabe.* Kössen: PM-Verlag, 2000.
4. Andreasen NC, Arndt S, Alliger R, et al. Symptoms of schizophrenia: methods, meanings, and mechanisms. *Arch Gen Psychiatry* 1995; **5**:341–51.
5. Möller HJ. Neuroleptic treatment of negative symptoms in schizophrenic patients. Efficacy problems and methodological difficulties. *Eur Neuropsychopharmacol* 1993; **3**:1–12.
6. Naber D, Holzbach R, Perro C, et al. Clinical management of clozapine patients in relation to efficacy and side effects. *Br J Psychiatry* 1992; **160**(Suppl.17):54–9.
7. Kane J, Honigfield G, Singer J, Meltzer H. Clozapine for the treatment-resistant schizophrenia: a double-blind comparison with chlorpromazine. *Arch Gen Psychiatry* 1988; **45**:789–96.
8. Emsley RA. Role of newer atypical antipsychotics in the management of treatment-resistant schizophrenia. *CNS Drugs* 2000; **13**:409–20.
9. Masand PS, Berry SL. Switching antipsychotic therapies. *Ann Pharmacother* 2000; **34**:200–7.

10. Wolkowitz OM, Rapaport MH, Pickar D. Benzodiazepine augmentation of neuroleptics. In: Angrist B, Schultz SC, eds. *The Neuroleptic Non-Responsive Patient: Characterization and treatment.* Washington DC: American Psychiatric Press, 1990:89–108.

11. Schultz SC, Kahn EM, Baker RW, Conley RR. Lithium and carbamazepine augmentation in treatment refractory schizophrenia. In: Angrist B, Schultz SC, eds. *The Neuroleptic Non-Responsive Patient: Characterization and treatment.* Washington DC: American Psychiatric Press, 1990:109–36.

12. Goff DC, Brotman AW, Waites M, et al. Trial of fluoxetine added to neuroleptics for treatment resistant schizophrenic patients. *Am J Psychiatry* 1990; **147**:492–4.

13. Arana GW, Goff DC, Friedman M, et al. Does carbamazepine-induced reduction of plasma haloperidol levels worsen psychotic symptoms? *Am J Psychiatry* 1986; **143**:650–1.

14. Siris SG, Bermanzohn PC, Gonzales A, et al. The use of antidepressants for negative symptoms in a subset of schizophrenic patients. *Psychopharmacol Bull* 1991; **27**:331–5.

15. Goldman MB, Luchins DJ. Intermittent therapy and tardive dyskinesia: a literature review. *Hosp Community Psychiatry* 1984; **35**:1215–19.

16. Kissling W, Kane JM, Barnes TRE, et al. *Guidelines for Neuroleptic Relapse Prevention in Schizophrenia: Toward a consensus view.* Berlin: Springer-Verlag, 1991.

# Pharmacotherapy of panic disorder

4

## Introduction

Panic attacks have been described for centuries, but the classification of panic disorder as a discrete illness is quite recent. The disorder first appeared in DSM-III only in 1980.[1] The cardinal feature of the disorder is a panic attack.

A panic attack begins suddenly, is characterized by intense fear or discomfort, and has at least four of several possible cardiac, respiratory, neurologic or gastrointestinal symptoms. The attack then subsides or abates spontaneously, often leaving the individual shaken and confused.

DSM-IV recognizes three types of panic attacks: unexpected (or uncued), situationally bound (cued) and situationally predisposed.[2] Unexpected attacks are truly spontaneous. Situationally bound episodes always follow a particular stimulus or cue, such as having to use an elevator. Situationally predisposed attacks may or may not occur after a particular stimulus, or may occur only after repeated exposure to the stimulus.

In order for a diagnosis of panic disorder to be made, three conditions must be met: the patient must experience recurrent, *unexpected* attacks; at least one of the attacks is followed by one month of persistent concern or anxiety over the possibility of additional attacks; and the patient exhibits a significant change in behaviour related to the attacks (Table 4.1).[3]

When the panic attacks are recurrent, the patient may begin to avoid situations perceived to precipitate panic attacks or situations where getting help could be very difficult. Over time, this avoidance may evolve into frank agoraphobia (Figure 4.1).

*Table 4.1* Diagnostic criteria for panic disorder.

| DSM-IV criteria for panic disorder (code 300.xx) |
| --- |

A. Recurrent unexpected panic attacks (see below)

B. At least one of the attacks has been followed by 1 month or more of the following:
   - persistent concern about having additional panic attacks
   - worry about the implications of the attack or its consequences
   - a significant change in behaviour related to the attacks

C. The panic attacks are not caused by a substance

D. The panic attacks are not better accounted for by another diagnosis

| DSM-IV criteria for panic attack symptoms |
| --- |

**Note** A panic attack is not a codable disorder, therefore the clinician must code the specific diagnosis in which the panic attack occurs

A discrete period of intense fear or discomfort, in which four or more of the following symptoms developed abruptly and reached a peak within 10 minutes:
   - palpitations, pounding heart, or accelerated heart rate
   - sweating
   - trembling or shaking
   - sensations of shortness of breath or smothering
   - feeling of choking
   - chest pain discomfort
   - nausea or abdominal distress
   - feeling dizzy, unsteady, light-headed or faint
   - derealization or depersonalization
   - fear of losing control or 'going crazy'
   - fear of dying
   - paresthesias
   - chills or hot flushes

| ICD-10 criteria for panic disorder (category F41) |
| --- |

A. The individual experiences recurrent panic attacks that are not consistently associated with a specific situation or object, and which often occur spontaneously (i.e. the episodes are unpredictable). The panic attacks are not associated with marked exertion or with exposure to dangerous or life-threatening situations

*Table 4.1* cont.

B. A panic attack is characterized by all of the following:
   (1) it is a discrete episode of intense fear or discomfort
   (2) it starts abruptly
   (3) it reaches a maximum within a few minutes and lasts at least some minutes
   (4) at least four of the symptoms listed below must be present, one of which must be from items (a)–(d):
   - Autonomic arousal symptoms:
     (a) palpitations or pounding heart, or accelerated heart rate
     (b) sweating
     (c) trembling or shaking
     (d) dry mouth (not due to medication or dehydration)
   - Symptoms involving chest and abdomen:
     (e) difficulty breathing
     (f) feeling of choking
     (g) chest pain or discomfort
     (h) nausea or abdominal distress, e.g. churning in stomach
   - Symptoms involving mental state:
     (i) feeling dizzy, unsteady, faint or light-headed
     (j) feelings that objects are unreal (derealization) or that the self is distant or 'not really here' (depersonalization)
     (k) fear of losing control, 'going crazy' or passing out
     (l) fear of dying
   - General symptoms:
     (m) hot flushes or cold chills
     (n) numbness or tingling sensations

C. Most commonly used exclusion clause: panic attacks are not due to a physical disorder, organic mental disorder (categories F00–F09) or other mental disorders such as schizophrenia and related disorders (F20–F29), mood [affective] disorders (F30–F39) or somatoform disorders (F45.x)
   The range of individual variation in both content and severity is so great that two grades, moderate and severe, may be specified, if desired, with a fifth character:
   F41.00    panic disorder, moderate (at least four panic attacks in a 4-week period)
   F41.01    panic disorder, severe (at least four panic attacks per week over a 4-week period)

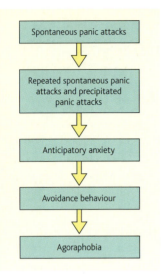

*Figure 4.1* Development of panic disorder.

Spontaneous panic attacks

Repeated spontaneous panic attacks and precipitated panic attacks

Anticipatory anxiety

Avoidance behaviour

Agoraphobia

In making the diagnosis of panic disorder, it is very important to confirm with the patient that *unexpected* panic attacks have occurred recurrently. The occurrence of other kinds of panic attack is associated with simple phobias, social anxiety disorder or other disorders.

Patients with panic disorder frequently present to primary care settings. In fact, estimates are that up to one in nine patients presenting for treatment in primary care centres suffer from panic disorder.[4] Such patients often complain of multiple general medical concerns. The differential diagnosis of panic disorder includes a variety of cardiac, endocrine, neurologic and respiratory disorders (Table 4.2).[5] The treatment decisions for panic disorder are shown in Figure 4.2.

## Decision 1: treatment of choice

Controlled trials have shown efficacy for several different agents in panic disorder, including certain high-potency benzodiazepines, tricyclic antidepressants, and selective serotonin reuptake inhibitors

**Table 4.2** *Differential diagnosis of panic disorder.*

| General medical illnesses | |
|---|---|
| • Anaemia | • Hypertension |
| • Angina | • Hyperthyroidism |
| • Arrhythmias | • Hypoglycaemia |
| • Cardiovascular disease | • Parathyroid disorders |
| • Chronic obstructive pulmonary disease | • Peptic ulcers |
| • Cushing's disease | • Pheochromocytoma |
| • Electrolyte disturbance | • Pulmonary embolus |
| • Epilepsy, particularly temporal attacks lobe epilepsy | • Transient ischaemic attacks |

(SSRIs).[6] There are fewer trials directly comparing the efficacy of different classes of medication, but meta-analysis has suggested that SSRIs may be more effective than older agents.[7]

Indeed, the SSRIs have emerged as the first-line pharmacotherapy of choice for panic disorder. They are not only effective, but also have a relatively benign side-effect profile, are safe and without dependence potential, and allow once-a-day dosing. Disadvantages include delayed onset of action, possible early anxiogenic effects, and sexual side effects. In panic disorder the efficacy of citalopram, escitalopram,[8] fluoxetine, fluvoxamine, paroxetine and sertraline has been documented in multicentre placebo-controlled clinical trials.[9]

Patients with panic disorder tend to be especially sensitive to side effects, and may experience an early increase in anxiety symptoms in response to antidepressant treatment.[10] It is therefore best to initiate therapy with low doses of antidepressants (e.g. citalopram 10 mg or paroxetine 10 mg). In general, antidepressant duration and dose required for efficacy in panic disorder are similar to those needed in major depression, although it is sometimes necessary to go higher. For paroxetine, for example, 40 mg was the lowest effective dose in one study.[11]

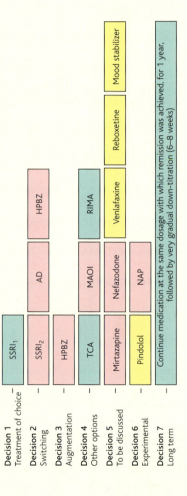

Key
AD = antidepressant; ECT = electroconvulsive therapy;
HPBZ = high-potency benzodiazepine; MAOI = monoamine oxidase inhibitor;
NAP = new generation antipsychotic; RIMA = reversible inhibitor of
monoamine oxidase type A; SSRI₁ = first selective serotonin reuptake inhibitor*;
SSRI₂ = second selective serotonin reuptake inhibitor*; TCA = tryciclic antidepressant

**Decision 1**
Treatment of choice — SSRI₁

**Decision 2**
Switching — SSRI₂ | AD | HPBZ

**Decision 3**
Augmentation — HPBZ

**Decision 4**
Other options — TCA | MAOI | RIMA

**Decision 5**
To be discussed — Mirtazapine | Nefazodone | Venlafaxine | Reboxetine | Mood stabilizer

**Decision 6**
Experimental — Pindolol | NAP

**Decision 7**
Long term — Continue medication at the same dosage with which remission was achieved, for 1 year, followed by very gradual down-titration (6–8 weeks)

Key (colour legend): ■ Intervention supported by consistent randomized trials ■ Intervention supported by limited controlled data ■ Intervention supported by uncontrolled data. (*SSRI₁ denotes treatment of choice; SSRI₂ suggests using a second SSRI after a therapeutic attempt with SSRI₁ has failed.)

**Figure 4.2** Treatment decisions for panic disorder.

While the focus of this volume is on pharmacotherapy, it should be emphasized that cognitive-behavioural interventions for panic disorder have also been shown effective.[12] There have been relatively few direct comparisons of these modalities or their optimal sequencing, and these studies are not always consistent;[13] nevertheless, from a clinical perspective it would be reasonable to incorporate CBT principles into the pharmacotherapeutic treatment of many patients.

## Comorbidity

Depression is frequently comorbid with panic disorder.[14] In such cases, despite the relative dearth of clinical trials focusing specifically on subjects with comorbid depression-panic, it seems rational to use medications with proven efficacy in both these disorders. In patients with comorbid substance abuse and in patients with personality disorders, although there is again a relative lack of relevant empirical studies, many clinicians would hold that benzodiazepines are not, in general, the first-line choice.[15]

## Baseline anxiety

Patients with high levels of baseline anxiety may benefit from initial treatment with benzodiazepines alone or benzodiazepines in combination with SSRIs, with subsequent discontinuation of benzodiazepines over several weeks. Certainly, meta-analysis of controlled trials of depression indicates that the combination of an antidepressant with a benzodiazepine has some benefits over the short term, although there are also possible risks to such an approach.[16]

# Decision 2: switching

Should a particular SSRI prove ineffective or poorly tolerated after a trial of adequate dose and duration, switching to a different medication can be considered. There are few studies focusing on panic disorder patients that have failed a first trial. The depression literature indicates that where one SSRI proves ineffective, another may prove useful,[17] and many would suggest that a similar principle holds true for panic disorder also. An alternative would, however, be to switch to an agent from an entirely different class.[18]

In the past, for example, the high-potency benzodiazepines (particularly, alprazolam and clonazepam) were considered a first-line treatment for panic disorder. They have the advantage of rapid onset and general anti-anxiety effects. They are also safe in overdose. However, ineffectiveness for comorbid depression, increasing concerns about side effects, including cognitive impairment and sedation, and problems with discontinuation have diminished their popularity.

Initial dosing of these agents should begin at 0.75–1.5 mg in divided doses for alprazolam and 0.25–0.5 mg for clonazepam (and comparable doses for other benzodiazepines) and should be titrated over a period of weeks to effective levels to obtain relief from panic symptoms (in the range of 3–4 mg/day for alprazolam and 1–2 mg/day for clonazepam).

Additional agents that can possibly be considered for treatment-refractory patients are briefly discussed at decision levels 4 through 6 below.

## Decision 3: augmentation

The question of when to switch and when to augment is one that has received little empirical study in panic disorder. One approach may, for example, be: to switch when there is no response or a partial response to the first trial; to switch or augment if there is a partial response to a second trial; and to augment when there is still no response to a third trial.

Unfortunately, the evidence base on augmentation strategies in panic disorder is also minimal. Given the efficacy of high-potency benzodiazepines in panic disorder, augmentation with one of these agents may, however, be considered in patients who have had a partial response to an SSRI or other antidepressant.[19]

# Decision 4: other options

Tricyclic antidepressants (TCAs) were the first medications shown to be efficacious for panic disorder.[7] For example, clomipramine, a particularly serotonergic TCA, is highly effective in panic disorder, and is widely used in Europe. Advantages include efficacy, antidepressant effects, no abuse potential and once-daily dosing. However, the less desirable side-effect profiles of many of the TCAs seldom make them a first choice of pharmacotherapy in panic disorder. Adverse effects of the TCAs include initial stimulation, anticholinergic effects, postural hypotension, sedation, sexual side effects and potential lethality in overdose.

Although not often studied in rigorous trials of panic disorder, the MAOIs have a reputation for being particularly effective in panic disorder. However, a problematic side-effect profile, together with the inconvenience of dietary restrictions and drug interactions, means that these agents are typically used only in refractory cases. RIMAs, such as moclobemide, on the other hand, have been shown useful in panic disorder and have an acceptable side-effect and interaction profile.

# Decision 5: treatments to be discussed

Although less well studied, a number of other medications can potentially be considered in patients with panic disorder. Several newer antidepressants, such as mirtazapine, nefazodone, venlafaxine and reboxetine may be useful in panic disorder.[20–22] Several mood stabilizers may also be effective in the treatment of panic disorder; these include gabapentin and valproate, although at this stage the data are very limited.[23]

# Decision 6: experimental

An interesting placebo-controlled study found that patients with treatment-resistant panic disorder responded to augmentation of fluoxetine with pindolol.[24] The new-generation antipsychotics have not been rigorously studied in panic disorder. Nevertheless, given their apparent efficacy in treatment-resistant depression, it would seem reasonable to consider their use in patients that proved refractory to usual treatments.

## Decision 7: long-term approach

Panic is a recurrent and often chronic disorder. In a four-year naturalistic follow-up of patients participating in a large multicentre trial, approximately one-third of patients had recovered and stayed well, while the remainder suffered from some remaining illness.[25] One in five patients reported a severe and chronic course. These findings suggest that treatment of panic disorder should be relatively long term. Indeed, current clinical consensus is that maintenance pharmacotherapy should be continued for at least a year.[6]

This recommendation is supported by a limited number of long-term placebo-controlled medication studies of panic disorder. In one study, patients were treated with paroxetine for 22 weeks, including 3 months of continued well status; then randomized to continuation on paroxetine or switched to placebo. Of those switched to placebo, nearly one-third had a recurrence, whereas only one in 20 of those on paroxetine suffered a recurrence.[26] In another, sertraline was superior to placebo in maintaining improvement and also well tolerated, in an 80-week treatment period.[27] Once the decision has been made to discontinue medication, a very gradual down-titration may be attempted (for example, decreasing 20–30% of the dose every few months).

## References

1. American Psychiatric Association. *Diagnostic and Statistical Manual of Mental Disorders*, 3rd edn. Washington DC: American Psychiatric Association, 1980.
2. American Psychiatric Association: *Diagnostic and Statistical Manual of Mental Disorders*, 4th edn. Washington DC: American Psychiatric Association, 1994.

3. Hirschfeld RMA. Panic disorder: diagnosis, epidemiology and clinical course. *J Clin Psychiatry* 1996; **57**(Suppl.10):3–8.

4. Shear MK, Schulberg JC. Anxiety disorders in primary care. *Bull Menninger Clin* 1995; **59**(2, Suppl.A):A73–A85.

5. Ballenger JC. Panic disorder in the medical setting. *J Clin Psychiatry* 1997; **58**(Suppl.2):13–17.

6. Ballenger JC, Davidson JRT, Lecrubier Y, et al. Consensus statement on panic disorder from the International Consensus Group on Depression and Anxiety. *J Clin Psychiatry* 1998; **59**(Suppl.):47–54.

7. Boyer W. Serotonin uptake inhibitors are superior to imipramine and alprazolam in alleviating panic attacks: A meta-analysis. *Int Clin Psychopharmacol* 1995; **10**:45–9.

8. Stahl SM, Gergel I, Li D. Escitalopram in the Treatment of Panic Disorder. Poster presentation at the 2002 American Psychiatric Association (APA) meeting, Philadelphia, PA, USA.

9. Bakker A, van Balkom AJ, van Dyck R. Selective serotonin reuptake inhibitors in the treatment of panic disorder and agoraphobia. *Int Clin Psychopharmacol* 2000; **15**(Suppl.):25–30.

10. Pohl R, Yergani VK, Balon Rea. The jitteriness syndrome in panic disorder patients treated with antidepressants. *J Clin Psychiatry* 1988; **49**:100–4.

11. Ballenger JC, Steiner M, Bushnell W, et al. Double-blind, fixed-dose, placebo-controlled study of paroxetine in the treatment of panic disorder. *Am J Psychiatry* 1998; **155**:36–42.

12. American Psychiatric Association. Practice guideline for the treatment of patients with panic disorder. *Am J Psychiatry* 1998; **155**:1–34.

13. Coplan JD, Gorman JM. Panic disorder. In: Fawcett J, Stein DJ, Jobson JO, eds. *Textbook of Treatment Algorithms in Psychopharmacology*. Chichester: John Wiley, 1999.

14. Roy-Byrne PP, Stang P, Wittchen H-U, et al. Lifetime panic-depression comorbidity in the National Comorbidity Survey: association with symptoms, impairment, course and help-seeking. *Br J Psychiatry* 2000; **176**:229–35.

15. Posternak MA, Mueller TI. Assessing the risks and benefits of benzodiazepines for anxiety disorders in patients with a history of substance abuse or dependence. *Am J Addict* 2000; **10**:48–68.

16. Furukawa TA, Streiner DL, Young LT. Antidepressant plus benzodiazepine for major depression (Cochrane Review). *Cochrane Database Syst Rev* 2001; **2**:CD001026.

17. Nelson JC. Augmentation strategies with serotonergic-noradrenergic combinations. *J Clin Psychiatry* 1998; **59**(Suppl.):65–8.

18. Tesar GE, Rosenbaum JF. Successful use of clonazepam in patients with treatment-resistant panic disorder. *J Nerv Ment Dis* 1986; **174**:477–82.

19. Tiffon L, Coplan JD, Papp LA, et al. Augmentation strategies with tricyclic or fluoxetine treatment in seven partially responsive panic disorder patients. *J Clin Psychiatry* 1994; **55**:66–9.

20. Bystritsky A, Rosen R, Suri R, Vapnik T. Pilot open-label study of nefazodone in panic disorder. *Depress Anxiety* 1999; **10**:137–9.

21. Versiani M, Cassano G, Perugi G, et al. Reboxetine, a selective norepinephrine reuptake inhibitor, is an effective and well-tolerated treatment for panic disorder. *J Clin Psychiatry* 2002; **63**:31–7.

22. Pollack MH, Worthington JJ 3rd, Otto MW, et al. Venlafaxine for panic disorder: results from a double-blind, placebo-controlled study. *Psychopharmacol Bull* 1996; **32**:667–70.

23. Pande AC, Pollack MH, Crockatt J, et al. Placebo-controlled study of gabapentin treatment of panic disorder. *J Clin Psychopharmacol* 2000; **20**:467–71.

24. Hirschmann S, Dannon PN, Iancu I, et al. Pindolol augmentation in patients with treatment-resistant panic disorder: a double-blind, placebo-controlled trial. *J Clin Psychopharmacol* 2000; **20**:556–9.

25. Katschnig H, Amering M, Stolk JM, Ballenger JC. Predictors of quality of life in a long-term follow-up study in panic disorder patients after a clinical drug trial. *Psychopharmacol Bull* 1996; **32**(1):149–55.

26. Lydiard RB, Steiner M, Burnham D, et al. Efficacy studies of paroxetine in panic disorder. *Psychopharmacol Bull* 1998; **34**:175–82.

27. Rapaport MH, Wolkow W, Rubin A, Hackett E, Pollack M, Ota KY. Sertraline treatment of panic disorder: results of a long-term study. *Acta Psychiatr Scand* 2001; **104**:289–98.

# Pharmacotherapy of social anxiety disorder

## Introduction

Individuals with social anxiety disorder (formerly described as social phobia) suffer from a fear of being scrutinized and subsequently embarrassed or humiliated in social encounters. This fear leads to the avoidance of a multitude of performance and interaction situations where the individual is being observed or evaluated by others. These individuals may have few friends, experience trouble with dating, drop out of school or reject promotions at work.[1]

Social anxiety disorder only received proper recognition recently, when it was disentangled from other 'phobic neuroses' by the DSM-IV.[2] In the past, many tended to regard it as 'shyness' or 'personality style', rather than as a disorder. However, with awareness of the significant impact of social anxiety disorder on function and on quality of life, there has to some extent been a change in attitude towards it.[3] Certainly, there is now a great deal of evidence that this disorder can be a severe and painful disability. This recognition has also fostered a great deal of research, both clinical and pre-clinical, which has in turn improved the therapeutic armamentarium currently at our disposal.[4]

As in the case of other anxiety disorders, such as panic disorder, secondary avoidance is a key factor in causing disability. Individuals with social anxiety disorder are less likely to graduate from college and are less likely to achieve professional success. More than 90% report occupational impairment, while 10% are unemployed. In addition, the disorder can interfere substantially with leisure activities.[5]

Given that consulting a physician is itself a social interaction likely to be feared and avoided, and that social anxiety disorder has only recently received recognition in classification systems, it is not surprising that the disorder has been greatly underdiagnosed. Large-scale epidemiological studies emphasize how prevalent this condition really is. Indeed, the National Comorbidity Survey (NCS), conducted in the USA, reported a lifetime prevalence of 13.3% and a 12-month prevalence of 7.8%.[6]

Unfortunately, one common way in which individuals with social anxiety disorder attempt to combat the fear associated with the disorder is with the use of alcohol, which puts them at increasing risk of developing secondary alcoholism. Other complications include the development of depression, other anxiety disorders and suicidal ideation. Use of alcohol to allay anxiety was found in 50% of patients, visits to mental health programmes in 35% and suicide attempts in about 15%.[7]

Given the early age of onset of social anxiety disorder (mean age of onset is 13 years, with most patients developing the disorder before the age of 25), and the chronic course of untreated social anxiety disorder, the importance of early diagnosis and treatment is paramount. Early intervention may hypothetically prevent subsequent comorbidity and improve long-term outcome (Figure 5.1).

The high comorbidity on the one hand, and considerable heterogeneity in the clinical presentation of social anxiety disorder on the other, may on occasion present a diagnostic challenge for the clinician. Nevertheless, a careful history and psychiatric evaluation typically allow for an accurate diagnosis to be made. Diagnostic criteria for social anxiety disorder, according to the DSM-IV, are presented in Table 5.1.

Social anxiety disorder may be classified into a number of subtypes, including generalized social anxiety disorder (in which there is a fear of most social situations) and performance anxiety (which is limited to anxiety concerning one or two situations). Public speaking is the social situation most commonly feared in community studies.[6] In clinical settings, however, many patients suffer from a more generalized form of social anxiety disorder (Table 5.2).

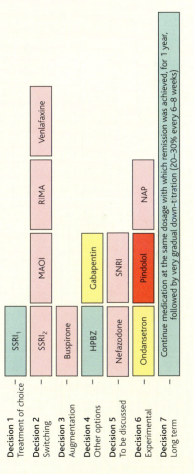

**Figure 5.1** *Treatment decisions for social anxiety disorder.* ■ *Intervention supported by consistent randomized trials* ■ *Intervention supported by limited controlled data* ■ *Intervention supported by uncontrolled data* ■ *Interventions that* ■ *have been found to be ineffective.* (*SSRI₁ denotes treatment of choice; SSRI₂ suggests using a second SSRI after a therapeutic attempt with SSRI₁ has failed.*)

Key
HPBZ = high potency benzodiazepines; MAOI = monoamine oxidase inhibitor; NAP = new generation antipsychotic; RIMA = reversible inhibitor of monoamine oxidase type A; SNRI = selective noradrenaline reuptake inhibitor; SSRI₁ = first selective serotonin reuptake inhibitor*; SSRI₂ = second selective serotonin reuptake inhibitor*; TCA = tryciclic antidepressant

**Decision 1** Treatment of choice — SSRI₁

**Decision 2** Switching — SSRI₂ | MAOI | RIMA | Venlafaxine

**Decision 3** Augmentation — Buspirone

**Decision 4** Other options — HPBZ | Gabapentin

**Decision 5** To be discussed — Nefazodone | SNRI

**Decision 6** Experimental — Ondansetron | Pindolol | NAP

**Decision 7** Long term — Continue medication at the same dosage with which remission was achieved, for 1 year, followed by very gradual down-titration (20–30% every 6–8 weeks)

*Table 5.1* *Diagnostic criteria for social anxiety disorder.*

| DSM-IV criteria for social anxiety disorder (code 300.23) |
| --- |
| A. A marked and persistent fear of one or more social or performance situations |
| B. Exposure to the feared social situation almost invariably provokes anxiety, which may take the form of a situationally bound or situationally predisposed panic attack |
| C. The person recognizes that the fear is excessive or unreasonable |
| D. The feared social or performance situations are avoided or are endured with intense anxiety or distress |
| E. The avoidance, anxious anticipation, or distress caused by the feared social or performance situation(s) interfere significantly with the person's normal routine, occupational/academic functioning, or social activities or relationships, or there is marked distress about having the phobia |
| F. The fear or avoidance is not caused by a substance or a general medical condition, and is not better accounted for by another mental disorder (e.g. panic disorder with or without agoraphobia, separation anxiety disorder, body dysmorphic disorder, a pervasive developmental disorder, or schizoid personality disorder) |

| ICD-10 criteria for social anxiety disorder (category F40.1) |
| --- |
| A. Fear of scrutiny by other people leading to avoidance of social situations |
| B. More pervasive social phobias usually associated with low self-esteem and fear of criticism |
| C. May present secondarily as a complaint of blushing, hand tremor, nausea or an urge to micturate |
| D. Patient can become convinced that one of these secondary manifestations is the primary problem |
| E. Symptoms may progress to panic attack |

*Table 5.2* *Social fears in the National Comorbidity Survey.*

| | | |
| --- | --- | --- |
| • Public speaking | • | Talking with others |
| • Using a toilet away from home | • | Writing while someone watches |
| • Eating or drinking in public | • | Talking in front of a small group |

# Decision 1: treatment of choice

## Social anxiety

Relatively few medication classes have proven effective in the treatment of social anxiety disorder, and there are few trials comparing different agents. Given the substantial evidence for their efficacy, safety and tolerability, the current consensus, however, is that SSRIs are the first-line pharmacotherapy of choice in social anxiety disorder.[4] Randomized controlled studies demonstrating the efficacy of SSRIs in treating social anxiety disorder include work with escitalopram, fluvoxamine, paroxetine and sertraline.[8]

An adequate trial of an SSRI in social anxiety disorder should be 10–12 weeks in duration.[4] Doses required for efficacy are similar to those needed in depression, although individual patients may require doses that approach maximally recommended doses.

While the focus of this volume is on pharmacotherapy, it should be emphasized that cognitive-behavioural interventions (CBT) for social anxiety disorder have also been shown effective. There have been relatively few direct comparisons of these modalities or their optimal sequencing, and these studies are not always consistent; nevertheless, from a clinical perspective, it would be reasonable to incorporate CBT principles into the pharmacotherapeutic treatment of many patients.[9]

## Performance anxiety

In patients with only limited performance anxiety, a beta-blocker may be useful.[10] Giving small doses of propranolol (40–80 mg), for example, about an hour before the performance, may help to alleviate tachycardia and other peripheral symptoms, preventing the snowball effect of anxiety resulting from awareness of these somatic symptoms.

It is, however, crucial not to miss the diagnosis of social anxiety disorder in patients who present with performance anxiety. SSRIs are effective not only in more generalized social anxiety disorder, but also in the less generalized variety.[11] In contrast, beta-blockers are ineffective for social anxiety disorder.

## Comorbidity

Depression is frequently comorbid with social anxiety disorder.[12] In such cases, despite the relative dearth of clinical trials focusing specifically on subjects with comorbid depression/social anxiety disorder, it seems rational to use medications with proven efficacy in both disorders. In patients with comorbid substance abuse and in patients with personality disorders, although there is again a relative lack of relevant empirical studies, many clinicians would hold that benzodiazepines are not, in general, the first-line choice.[13]

# Decision 2: switching

In the case that the individual with social anxiety disorder is not responding to an SSRI, there are two alternatives. One is to switch to another SSRI; the other is to utilize a medication with an entirely different mechanism of action (e.g. MAOIs or RIMAs). There are few empirical data on which to base this choice, although the literature on depression emphasizes that many patients who do not respond to one SSRI will respond to another.[14] Furthermore, there is an anecdotal literature suggesting that patients with social anxiety disorder who fail to respond to an SSRI may respond to venlafaxine, an agent with predominantly serotonergic reuptake inhibition at lower doses.[15]

Among the irreversible MAOIs, phenelzine is the most extensively studied, and its efficacy is well established.[10] Tranylcypromine is also effective in social anxiety disorder, although fewer data are available. From a clinical perspective, treatment with these irreversible MAOIs involves a relatively unfavourable side-effect profile, a restricted (tyramine-free) diet to avoid hypertensive crises, and close supervision of any concomitant medications (to prevent serious drug–drug interactions). Hence, despite their proven efficacy in social anxiety disorder, MAOIs are typically prescribed only when a number of other medications have failed. When switching from an SSRI to a MAOI, a wash-out period is required.

The reversible inhibitors of monoamine oxidase (RIMAs), such as moclobemide, have a favourable side-effect and drug interaction profile. At the standard dosage of 600 mg/day, moclobemide does not require dietary constraints. However, despite the initially encouraging results with the use of this compound in social anxiety disorder,[16] lately there has been some concern about its efficacy, based on more recent studies that have shown disappointing results.[17] Similarly, meta-analysis of the social anxiety disorder trials indicates that the effect size of the SSRIs is larger than that of the RIMAs,[8] arguably supporting a clinical decision to switch to a different SSRI rather than to a RIMA.

# Decision 3: augmentation

The question of when to switch and when to augment is one that has received little empirical study in social anxiety disorder. One approach may, for example, be to switch when there is no response or a partial response to the first trial, to switch or augment if there is a partial response to a second trial, and to augment when there is still no response to a third trial.

Furthermore, there is a paucity of evidence on the value of augmentation strategies in social anxiety disorder. Buspirone, a $5HT_{1A}$ partial agonist, was found ineffective when used as monotherapy for social anxiety disorder,[18] but may offer some value when used to augment an SSRI.[19]

# Decision 4: other options

Clonazepam was found effective in a randomized controlled trial of social anxiety disorder.[16] The medication reduced performance anxiety, avoidance, interpersonal sensitivity, fears of negative evaluation and disability. Moreover, two-year follow-up data suggested that a beneficial effect was maintained.

However, benzodiazepines are ineffective for comorbid depression and may not be advisable in patients with comorbid substance abuse. In addition, chronic use of benzodiazepines raises concerns about side effects such as cognitive impairment and sedation, and about potential difficulties in discontinuing medication. We have therefore placed this class of medication relatively low in our algorithm.

Gabapentin was found effective in a randomized controlled trial of social anxiety disorder.[20] Nevertheless, it is unclear whether this agent or other anticonvulsants will prove to have as robust an effect on symptoms as the SSRIs and benzodiazepines.

# Decision 5: treatments to be discussed

The role of newer antidepressants such as nefazodone and the SNRIs in social anxiety disorder has not been established in controlled trials.[4] However, uncontrolled studies have found venlafaxine to be effective in social anxiety disorder,[15] and this agent certainly deserves additional study.

# Decision 6: experimental approaches

The 5HT₃ antagonist, ondansentron, has been reported to be effective in social anxiety disorder in one preliminary 10-week study.[21] Further study is needed before this agent can be recommended.

Emerging data about the value of pindolol augmentation in enhancing serotonergic neurotransmission have increased interest in this agent. However, a controlled study of pindolol augmentation in social anxiety disorder was negative.[22]

The new generation antipsychotics have been found effective as augmenting agents in some mood and anxiety disorders. Nevertheless, these agents have also been associated with the exacerbation of social anxiety symptoms.[23]

# Decision 7: long-term approach

Although relatively little is known about the natural course of social anxiety disorder, recent epidemiological data suggest that generalized social anxiety disorder, which is the more severe form of the disorder, has a chronic and long-term course.[3–6] Current clinical consensus is that once significant improvement has been attained, patients should be maintained on medication for at least 1 year.[4]

A number of controlled studies of maintenance pharmacotherapy in social anxiety disorder support this recommendation. Once the decision has been made to discontinue medication, a very gradual down-titration may be attempted (for example, decreasing 20–30% of the dose every few months).

# References

1. Liebowitz MR, Gorman JM, Fryer A, et al. Social phobia: review of a neglected anxiety disorder. *Arch Gen Psychiatry* 1985; **42**:729–37.
2. American Psychiatric Association. *Diagnostic and Statistical Manual of Mental Disorders* (DSM-IV), 4th edn. Washington, DC: American Psychiatric Association, 1994.
3. Moutier CY, Stein MB. The history, epidemiology, and differential diagnosis of social anxiety disorder. *J Clin Psychiatry* 1999; **60**:4–8.
4. Ballenger JC, Davidson JA, Lecrubier Y, et al. Consensus statement on social anxiety disorder from the international consensus group on depression and anxiety. *J Clin Psychiatry* 1998; **59**:54–60.
5. Lopez-Ibor JJ Jr, Ayuso Gutierrez JL. Social phobia: a debilitating disease that needs treatment. *Int Clin Psychopharmacol* 1997; **12**:S11–S16.
6. Magee WJ, Eaton WW, Wittchen HU, et al. Agoraphobia, simple phobia, and social phobia in the National Comorbidity Survey. *Arch Gen Psychiatry* 1996; **53**:159–68.
7. Weiller E, Bisserbe J-C, Boyer P, et al. Social phobia in general healthcare. *Br J Psychiatry* 1996; **168**:169–74
8. van der Linden GJH, Stein DJ, van Balkom AJLM. The efficacy of the selective serotonin reuptake inhibitors for social anxiety disorder (social phobia): A meta-analysis of randomized controlled trials. *Int Clin Psychopharmacol* 2000; **15**(Suppl.2):15–24.
9. Sutherland SM, Davidson JRT. Social phobia. In: Fawcett J, Stein DJ, Jobson KO, eds. *Textbook of Treatment Algorithms in Psychopharmacology*. Chichester: John Wiley, 1999.
10. Liebowitz MR, Schneier FR, Campeas R, et al. Phenelzine vs. atenolol in social phobia: a placebo-controlled experiment. *Arch Gen Psychiatry* 1992; **49**:290–300.

11. Stein DJ, Stein MB, Goodwin W, et al. The selective serotonin reuptake inhibitor paroxetine is effective in more generalized and less generalized social anxiety disorder. *Psychopharmacology (Berl)* 2001; **158**(3):267–72.

12. Kessler RC, Stang P, Wittchen H-U, et al. Lifetime co-morbidities between social phobia and mood disorders in the US National Comorbidity Survey. *Psychol Med* 1999; **29**:555–67.

13. Posternak MA, Mueller TI. Assessing the risks and benefits of benzodiazepines for anxiety disorders in patients with a history of substance abuse or dependence. *Am J Addict* 2000; **10**:48-68.

14. Nelson JC. Treatment of antidepressant nonresponders: augmentation or switch. *J Clin Psychiatry* 1998; **59**(Suppl.):35–41.

15. Altamura AC, Pioli R, Vitto M, et al. Venlafaxine in social phobia: a study in selective serotonin reuptake non-responders. *Int Clin Psychopharmacol* 1999; **14**:239–45.

16. Versiani M, Nardi AE, Mundim FD, et al. Pharmacotherapy of social phobia: a controlled study with moclobemide and phenelzine. *Br J Psychiatry* 1992; **161**:353–60.

17. Noyes R Jr, Moroz G, Davidson JR, et al. Moclobemide in social phobia: a controlled dose–response trial. *J Clin Psychopharmacol* 1997; **17**:247–54.

18. van Vliet IM, den Boer JA, Westenberg HG, Pian KL. Clinical effects of buspirone in social phobia: a double-blind placebo-controlled study. *J Clin Psychiatry* 1997; **58**(4):164–8.

19. Van Ameringen M, Mancini C, Wilson C. Buspirone augmentation of selective serotonin reuptake inhibitors (SSRIs) in social phobia. *J Affect Disord* 1996; **39**:115–21.

20. Pande AC, Davidson JR, Jefferson JW, et al. Treatment of social phobia with gabapentin: a placebo-controlled study. *J Clin Psychopharmacol* 1999; **19**:341–8.

21. Bell J, DeVaugh-Geiss J. Multi-center trial of a 5-HT3 antagonist, ondansetron, in social phobia. Presented at the 33rd Annual Meeting of the American College of Neuropsychopharmacology; December 13, 1994; San Juan, Puerto Rico.

22. Stein MB, Sareen J, Hami S, et al. Pindolol potentiation of paroxetine for generalized social phobia: a double-blind, placebo-controllled, crossover study. *Am J Psychiatry* 2001; **158**:1725–7.

23. Pallanti S, Quercioli L, Rossi A, et al. The emergence of social phobia during clozapine treatment and its response to fluoxetine augmentation. *J Clin Psychiatry* 1999; **60**:819–23.

# Pharmacotherapy of post-traumatic stress disorder

6

## Introduction

In the past, post-traumatic stress disorder was primarily associated with combat-related events. This was reflected in the names given to the disorder – 'shell shock', 'soldier's heart', 'combat neurosis' and 'operational fatigue'.[1] In the late 1980s, it was realized that PTSD could be related to all types of traumatic events, such as rape, physical assault, a severe automobile accident and natural or man-made disasters. Consequently, the terms for the disorder were changed to 'traumatic neurosis' and later to 'PTSD'.[2]

The tendency to interpret the symptoms of what we would now consider PTSD – as a 'normal response' to traumatic events – was another factor that impeded progress in the field. It is important to emphasize that the majority of individuals who are exposed to a traumatic event will later adapt and continue normally with their lives. Only a relatively small percentage of those exposed to traumatic events develop the dysfunctional response of PTSD.[3]

A third factor that has been an obstacle in the recognition of PTSD as a 'real' diagnosis is the close linkage between the disorder and forensic issues. By definition, PTSD involves an internal response to an external event and there is therefore a possibility of litigation. It is perhaps not surprising that a differential diagnosis between PTSD and 'compensation neurosis' is often raised, although, based on epidemiological data, it appears that the majority of PTSD patients do not misrepresent their symptoms.[4]

It has been estimated that approximately one-third of the population will be exposed to a severe trauma during their lifetime.[3] Since 10–20% of individuals exposed to severe trauma will develop

PTSD, the prevalence of PTSD in the general population will be in the range of 3–6%. This estimation has been confirmed in two studies carried out in the USA.[5,6] However, most patients are not diagnosed and are, consequently, not treated. Figure 6.1 shows the time course of PTSD and its subtypes.

There are four characteristic features of PTSD:

- exposure to a traumatic event
- re-experiencing symptoms
- avoidance/numbing
- increased arousal.

According to the DSM-IV (Table 6.1), the classification of a traumatic event only includes exposure to a situation where 'the person experienced, witnessed, or was confronted with an event or events that involved actual or threatened death or serious injury, or a threat to physical integrity of self or others'.[7] According to this definition, very severe humiliation, or any other type of disappointment or intense stress, does not fulfil the criteria for a traumatic event.

The second feature of PTSD is re-experiencing the traumatic event. For individuals with the disorder, it is as if the clock stopped at the time of the trauma, and from this time onward they often re-live these events in the form of intrusive memories, flashbacks and nightmares.

One of the maladaptive mechanisms used by patients with anxiety disorders is *avoidance* – the third feature of PTSD. PTSD sufferers attempt to avoid any stimuli associated with the trauma and also show markedly diminished interest in usual activities. It is believed that this 'emotional anaesthesia' or numbing is yet another maladaptive component of persistent avoidance.

The fourth feature of PTSD is increased arousal. Patients are constantly 'on alert', have difficulty in falling or staying asleep, suffer from irritability or outbursts of anger, have difficulty concentrating and experience hypervigilance and exaggerated startle response.

In addition to the type and magnitude of the trauma, high-risk factors for PTSD include personal characteristics such as high neuroticism scores, pre-existing depression and anxiety, lower level of education and earlier exposure to traumatic events (childhood separation from parents, childhood abuse, sexual assault and parental divorce in early childhood).

**Table 6.1** *Diagnostic criteria for post-traumatic stress disorder (PTSD).*

| DSM-IV criteria for PTSD (code 309.81) |
| --- |

A.  The person has been exposed to a traumatic event in which both of the following were present:
   (1) the person experienced, witnessed, or was confronted with an event or events that involved actual or threatened death or serious injury, or a threat to the physical integrity of self or others
   (2) the person's response involved intense fear, helplessness, or horror. (In children this may be expressed by disorganized or agitated behaviour)

B.  The traumatic event is persistently re-experienced in at least one of the following ways:
   (1) recurrent and intrusive distressing recollections of the event, including images, thoughts or perceptions. (In children, repetitive play may occur in which themes or aspects of the trauma are expressed)
   (2) recurrent distressing dreams of the event. (In children there may be frightening dreams without recognizable content)
   (3) acting or feeling as if the traumatic event were recurring (such as a sense of re-living the experience, illusions, hallucinations and dissociative flashback episodes, including those that occur on awakening or when intoxicated). (In children trauma-specific re-enactment may occur)
   (4) intense psychological distress or exposure to internal or external cues that symbolize or resemble an aspect of the traumatic event
   (5) physiological reactivity on exposure to internal or external cues that symbolize or resemble an aspect of the traumatic event

C.  Persistent avoidance of stimuli associated with the trauma and numbing of general responsiveness (not present before the trauma) as shown by three or more of the following:
   (1) efforts to avoid thoughts, feelings, or conversations associated with the trauma

*cont.*

*Table 6.1* cont.

(2) efforts to avoid activities, places, or people that arouse memories of the trauma

(3) inability to recall an important aspect of the trauma

(4) markedly diminished interest or participation in significant activities

(5) feeling of detachment or estrangement from others

(6) restricted range of affect (e.g. unable to have loving feelings)

(7) sense of a foreshortened future (e.g. does not expect to have a career, marriage, children, or a normal life span)

D. Persistent symptoms of increased arousal (not present before the trauma) as shown by two or more of the following:

(1) difficulty falling or staying asleep

(2) irritability or outbursts of anger

(3) difficulty concentrating

(4) hypervigilance

(5) exaggerated startle response

E. Duration of the disturbance (symptoms in B, C, and D) is more than 1 month

F. Disturbance causes clinically significant distress or impairment in social, occupational, or other important areas of functioning

*Note*

- PTSD is **acute** if symptoms last less than 3 months
- PTSD is **chronic** if symptoms last 3 months or more
- PTSD is with **delayed onset** if onset of symptoms is at least 6 months after the trauma

**ICD-10 criteria for PTSD (category F43.1)**

A. Arises as a delayed or protracted response to a stressful event or situation (of either short or long duration) of an exceptionally threatening or catastrophic nature, which is likely to cause pervasive distress in almost anyone. Predisposing factors such as personality traits (e.g. compulsive, asthenic) or previous history of neurotic illness, may lower the threshold for the development of the syndrome or aggravate its course, but they are neither necessary nor sufficient to explain its occurrence

B. Typical features include:

- episodes of repeated re-living of the trauma in intrusive memories ('flashbacks'), dreams or nightmares occurring against the persisting background of a sense of numbness and emotional blunting

*Table 6.1*  cont.

|  | • detachment from other people |
|--|--|
|  | • unresponsiveness to surroundings |
|  | • anhedonia |
|  | • avoidance of activities and situations reminiscent of the trauma |
| C. | Usually a state of autonomic hyperarousal with hypervigilance, an enhanced startle reaction, and insomnia |
| D. | Anxiety and depression are commonly associated with any of the above, and suicidal ideation is not infrequent |

*Note*
- Onset of PTSD follows the trauma with a latency period of a few weeks to a few months
- The course is fluctuating but recovery can be expected in most cases
- In a few cases the condition may follow a chronic course over many years, with eventual transition to an enduring personality change (category F62.0)

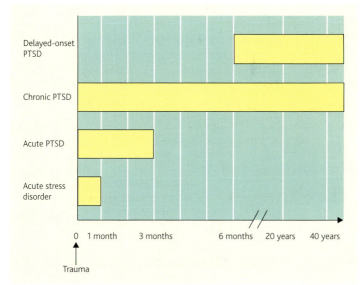

*Figure 6.1*  *Time course of PTSD and subtypes.*

# Decision 1: treatment of choice

Controlled trials have shown efficacy for several different agents in PTSD, including SSRIs, TCAs, and MAOIs. There are fewer trials directly comparing the efficacy of different classes of medication, but given the substantial evidence for their efficacy, safety and tolerability, the current consensus is that SSRIs are the first-line pharmacotherapy of choice in PTSD (Figure 6.2).[8,9] Controlled studies have been undertaken with fluoxetine, paroxetine and sertraline, and there are open trials with citalopram and fluvoxamine.[8] These agents are clearly effective in civilian PTSD, and although the evidence is more conflicting, may also be effective in combat PTSD.[10]

Careful evaluation of symptoms prior to treatment will allow therapeutic effects on target symptoms to be assessed systematically. An adequate trial of an SSRI in PTSD should be 10–12 weeks in duration.[9] Doses required for efficacy may be similar to those needed in depression, although individual patients may require maximally recommended doses.

While the focus of this volume is on pharmacotherapy, it should be emphasized that cognitive-behavioural (CBT) interventions for PTSD have long been shown effective. There have been few direct comparisons of pharmacotherapy and psychotherapy or their optimal sequencing; nevertheless, from a clinical perspective it would be reasonable to incorporate CBT principles into the pharmacotherapeutic treatment of many patients.[11,12]

# Decision 2: switching

If the patient is not tolerating or responding to an SSRI, a different agent may be considered. There are few empirical data on which to base this choice, although the literature on depression emphasizes that many patients who do not respond to one SSRI will respond to another.[13] Indeed, nefazodone, which has serotonin reuptake properties, was found effective in an open-label case series of treatment-refractory PTSD.[14]

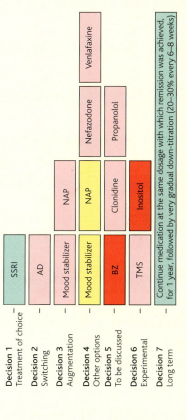

**Figure 6.2** Treatment decisions for PTSD. ■ *Intervention supported by consistent randomized trials* ■ *Intervention supported by limited controlled data* ■ *Intervention supported by uncontrolled data* ■ *Interventions that have been found to be ineffective.*

Key
AD = antidepressant;
BZ = benzodiazepine;
NAP = new generation antipsychotic;
SSRI = selective serotonin reuptake inhibitor;
TMS = transcranial magnetic stimulation

| | | | |
|---|---|---|---|
| **Decision 1** Treatment of choice | SSRI | | |
| **Decision 2** Switching | AD | | |
| **Decision 3** Augmentation | Mood stabilizer | NAP | |
| **Decision 4** Other options | Mood stabilizer | NAP | |
| **Decision 5** To be discussed | BZ | Clonidine | Propanolol |
| **Decision 6** Experimental | TMS | Inositol | |
| **Decision 7** Long term | Continue medication at the same dosage with which remission was achieved, for 1 year, followed by very gradual down-titration (20–30% every 6–8 weeks) | | |

Nefazodone / Venlafaxine (Decision 4 row)

TCAs (amitriptyline and imipramine) have also been shown effective in controlled studies of PTSD. Doses used were: amitriptyline 150–250 mg[15] and a mean dose of imipramine 225 mg.[16] However, given the relatively unfavourable side-effect profiles of these agents, TCAs are less popular for PTSD than in the past. Caution may be necessary when switching from an SSRI to a TCA, particularly when the SSRI has a long half-life and inhibits cytochrome P450 enzymes.

In a comparative study of phenelzine versus imipramine for PTSD, phenelzine was more effective for some symptom clusters than imipramine.[16] However, the side-effect profile, dietary restrictions (i.e. a low tyramine diet) and drug–drug interactions associated with this medication limit its use in a disorder where impulsivity may be problematic. When switching from an SSRI to a MAOI a wash-out period is required.

# Decision 3: augmentation

The question of when to switch and when to augment is one that has received little empirical study in PTSD. One approach may, for example, be to switch when there is no or partial response to the first trial, to switch or augment if there is a partial response to a second trial, and to augment when there is still no response to a third trial. Unfortunately, there are few controlled studies of medication augmentation in PTSD.[17]

Given the multiple symptoms of PTSD, another approach is to add medications that speculatively target specific symptom types. For example, in PTSD patients where anger outbursts are problematic, a mood stabilizer such as lithium or an anticonvulsant could be tried. Several of these agents have proven effective in uncontrolled studies of PTSD, although only lamotrigine has been studied as monotherapy in a controlled trial.[17]

Similarly, in PTSD patients where agitation is a problem, low doses of a new generation antipsychotic may be added. There is a small anecdotal literature on the use of the older antipsychotics in PTSD; the newer generation agents have a more favourable side-effect profile, and some of these agents have recently been investigated as monotherapy.[18]

# Decision 4: other options

As noted earlier, there is some evidence that various mood stabilizers and new generation antipsychotics may be useful as monotherapy in PTSD. Anecdotal evidence exists for the value of lithium, valproate, carbamazepine, and some traditional antipsychotics in treating this disorder.[19] There is preliminary controlled evidence for the efficacy of lamotrigine and risperidone in particular.

Nefazodone has been reported to be effective in some uncontrolled work on PTSD.[20] Controlled studies of this agent have been undertaken, but the data remain unpublished. Venlafaxine, which is predominantly a serotonin reuptake inhibitor at lower doses, may be hypothesized to be effective in PTSD, and deserves rigorous study.

# Decision 5: treatment to be discussed

There is little evidence for the efficacy of benzodiazepines in the treatment of PTSD.[21] In one study, there was even a suggestion that administration of alprazolam after trauma was associated with an increased risk for the development of PTSD.[22] Taken together with the various known disadvantages of benzodiazepines, this work suggests caution in using these agents for PTSD.[23]

Various adrenergic agents, including clonidine, an $\alpha_2$ adrenergic agonist, and propranolol (a beta-blocker) have been reported effective in uncontrolled studies of PTSD.[19] These agents deserve further controlled investigation in this condition.

# Decision 6: experimental approaches

Although TMS has been attempted with a few PTSD patients with promising results, further studies are needed to determine whether this technique has a role in the disorder.[24]

One double-blind study with inositol found no difference from placebo in PTSD.[25] This study was, however, limited by its short duration.

# Decision 7: long-term approach

Very little is known about the natural course of PTSD and even less is known about maintenance treatment. It seems, however, that in most cases there is a spontaneous decrease in the symptoms of PTSD in the first 6 months following the trauma, which continues for up to 4 years or longer.[6] From this standpoint, one should take into account the possibility of spontaneous recovery when prescribing medication at different time intervals after trauma.

For patients who clearly have PTSD that is of chronic duration, long-term administration of medication may, however, be required. Current clinical consensus indicates that medication should be continued for at least a year after acute treatment response.[9] Once a decision is made to discontinue medication, a general clinical rule for the anxiety disorders is to taper medication very slowly (for example, decreasing 20–30% of the dose every few months). A special consideration in the maintenance treatment of patients with PTSD is exacerbation of symptoms on specific dates in the year, such as the anniversary of the trauma, or memorial days for veterans. Although there is little published literature on the pharmacotherapy of such PTSD exacerbations, careful monitoring may be appropriate, with possible increase in medication dosage where needed.

# References

1. Yehuda R, McFarlane AC. Conflict between current knowledge about posttraumatic stress disorder and its original conceptual basis. *Am J Psychiatry* 1995; **152**:1705–13.
2. American Psychiatric Association. *Diagnostic and Statistical Manual of Mental Disorders* (DSM-III), 3rd edn. Washington, DC: American Psychiatric Association, 1980.

3. Breslau N, Davis GC, Andreski P. Traumatic events and posttraumatic stress disorder in an urban population of young adults. *Arch Gen Psychiatry* 1991; **48**:216–22.

4. Hales RE, Zatzick DF. What is PTSD? *Am J Psychiatry* 1997; **154**:143–5.

5. Breslau N, Kessler RC, Chilcoat HD, et al. Trauma and posttraumatic stress disorder in the community: The 1996 Detroit Area Survey of Trauma. *Arch Gen Psychiatry* 1996; **55**:626–32.

6. Kessler RC, Sonnega A, Bromet E, et al. Posttraumatic stress disorder in the National Comorbidity Survey. *Arch Gen Psychiatry* 1995; **52**:1048–60.

7. American Psychiatric Association. *Diagnostic and Statistical Manual of Mental Disorders* (DSM-IV), 4th edn. Washington, DC: American Psychiatric Association, 1994.

8. Stein DJ, Zungu-Dirwayi N, van der Linden GJ, et al. Pharmacotherapy for posttraumatic stress disorder. *Cochrane Database of Systematic Reviews* 2000; **4**:CD002795.

9. Ballenger JC, Davidson JR, Lecrubier Y, et al. Consensus statement on posttraumatic stress disorder from the International Consensus Group on Depression and Anxiety. *J Clin Psychiatry* 2000; **61**(Suppl.5):60–6.

10. Zohar J, Amital D, Miodownik C, et al. Double-blind placebo-controlled pilot study of sertraline in military veterans with posttraumatic stress disorder. *J Clin Psychopharmacol* 2002; **22**(2):190–5.

11. Marshall RD, Yehuda R, Liebowitz MR. Post-traumatic stress disorder. In: Fawcett J, Stein, DJ, Jobson, KO, eds. *Textbook of Treatment Algorithms in Psychopharmacology*. Chichester: John Wiley, 1999.

12. Southwick SM, Yehuda R. The interaction between pharmacotherapy and psychotherapy in the treatment of posttraumatic stress disorder. *Am J Psychotherapy* 1993; **47**:404–11.

13. Nelson JC. Treatment of antidepressant nonresponders: augmentation or switch? *J Clin Psychiatry* 1998; **59**(Suppl.15):35–41.

14. Zisook S, Chentsova-Dutton YE, Smith-Vaniz A, et al. Nefazodone in patients with treatment-refractory posttraumatic stress disorder. *J Clin Psychiatry* 2000; **61**:203–8.

15. Davidson J, Kudler H, Smith R, et al. Treatment of posttraumatic stress disorder with amitriptyline and placebo. *Arch Gen Psychiatry* 1990; **47**:259–66.

16. Kosten TR, Frank JB, Dan E, et al. Pharmacotherapy for posttraumatic stress disorder using phenelzine or imipramine. *J Nerv Ment Dis* 1991; **179**:366–70.

17. Hertzberg MA, Butterfield M, I, Feldman ME, et al. A preliminary study of lamotrigine for the treatment of posttraumatic stress disorder. *Biol Psychiatry* 1999; **45**:1226–9.
18. Leyba CM, Wampler TP. Risperidone in PTSD. *Psychiatr Serv* 1998; **49**:245–6.
19. Davison JRT. Biological therapies for posttraumatic stress disorder: an overview. *J Clin Psychiatry* 1997; **58**:29–32.
20. Davidson JRT, Weisler RH, Malik ML, Connor MK. Treatment of posttraumatic stress disorder with nefazodone. *Int Clin Psychopharmacol* 1998; **13**:111–13.
21. Braun P, Greenberg D, Dasberg H, et al. Core symptoms of posttraumatic stress disorder unimproved by alprazolam treatment. *J Clin Psychiatry* 1990; **51**:236–8.
22. Gelpin E, Bonne E, Peri T, et al. Treatment of recent trauma survivors with benzodiazepines: a prospective study. *J Clin Psychiatry* 1996; **57**:390–4.
23. Risse SC, Whitters A, Burke J, et al. Severe withdrawal symptoms after discontinuation of alprazolam in eight patients with combat-induced posttraumatic stress disorder. *J Clin Psychiatry* 1990; **51**:206–9.
24. Grisaru N, Amir M, Cohen H, et al. Effect of transcranial magnetic stimulation in posttraumatic stress disorder: a preliminary study. *Biol Psychiatry* 1998; **44**:52–5.
25. Kaplan Z, Amir M, Swartz M, et al. Inositol treatment of post-traumatic stress disorder. *Anxiety* 1996; **2**:51–2.

# Pharmacotherapy of obsessive-compulsive disorder

7

## Introduction

Once regarded as a rare illness of psychodynamic origin, OCD is now believed to be a rather common neuropsychiatric disorder affecting approximately 2% of the population.[1] OCD is characterized by intrusive, persistent, unwanted thoughts or images (obsessions) and by repetitive and excessive behaviours or mental acts (compulsions). The ego-dystonic nature of OCD is one of the hallmarks of this disorder, which is also associated with significant social and occupational impairment (Table 7.1).

The introduction of clomipramine (CMI) in the 1960s, and of the SSRIs in the late 1980s and early 1990s, has markedly improved the prognosis of patients with this disorder. Whereas OCD was once regarded as refractory to treatment, each of these serotonin reuptake inhibitors (SRIs) is associated with a response rate of around 40–60%.[2] Although our focus in this volume is on adults, it is notable that these agents have also been shown effective in paediatric OCD.[3] Further, the efficacy of serotonergic drugs in OCD has helped pave the way towards a better understanding of the pathophysiology of this disorder.[4,5]

It should also be emphasized that individual and family-based cognitive-behavioural (CBT) interventions for OCD have long been shown effective.[6] There have been relatively few direct comparisons of pharmacotherapy and psychotherapy or their optimal sequencing, and these studies are not always consistent; nevertheless, from a clinical perspective it would reasonable to incorporate CBT principles into the pharmacotherapeutic treatment of many patients (Figure 7.1).[7]

*Table 7.1* *Diagnostic criteria for obsessive-compulsive disorder (OCD)*

| DSM-IV criteria for OCD (code 300.3) |
| --- |
| A. Either obsessions or compulsions<br>Obsessions as defined by (1), (2), (3) and (4):<br>(1) recurrent and persistent thoughts, impulses or images<br>(2) the thoughts, impulses or images are not simply excessive worries about real life problems<br>(3) the person attempts to ignore, neutralize or suppress such thoughts, impulses or images<br>(4) the person recognizes that the obsessional thoughts, impulses or images are a product of his or her own mind not imposed externally, as in thought insertion<br>Compulsions as defined by (1) and (2):<br>(1) repetitive behaviours (e.g. hand washing, ordering and/or checking) or mental acts (e.g. praying, counting and/or repeating words silently) that the person feels driven to perform<br>(2) the behaviours or mental acts are aimed at preventing or reducing distress or preventing some dreaded event or situation |
| B. At some point during the course of the disorder, the person has recognized that the obsessions or compulsions are excessive or unreasonable (Note: this does not apply to children) |
| C. The obsessions or compulsions cause marked distress, are time consuming (take more than 1 hour a day) or significantly interfere with the person's normal routine |
| D. If another Axis I disorder is present, the content of the obsessions or compulsions is not restricted to it (e.g. preoccupation with food in the presence of an eating disorder; ruminations in the presence of major depressive disorder) |
| E. The disturbance is not a result of the direct physiological effects of a substance (e.g. a drug of abuse and/or a medication) or a general medical condition<br>*Definition*<br>With poor insight: If, for most of the time during the current episode, the person does not recognize that the obsessions and compulsions are excessive or unreasonable |

*Table 7.1* cont.

| ICD-10 criteria for OCD (category F42) |
| --- |
| A. Recurrent obsessional thoughts or compulsive acts: <br>  • obsessional thoughts are ideas, images or impulses that enter the patient's mind repeatedly in a stereotyped form. They are almost invariably distressing and the patient often tries, unsuccessfully, to resist them. They are recognized as the patient's own thoughts even though they are involuntary and often repugnant <br>  • compulsive acts or rituals are repeated stereotyped behaviours. They are not inherently enjoyable nor do they result in the completion of inherently useful tasks. Their function is to prevent some objectively unlikely event, often involving harm to or caused by the patient. This behaviour is recognized by the patient as pointless and repeated attempts are made to resist. Anxiety is nearly always present. If compulsive acts are resisted, the anxiety gets worse |
| B. OCD **includes** anankastic neurosis and obsessive-compulsive neurosis |
| C. OCD **excludes** obsessive-compulsive personality disorder (category F60.5) |
| D. Most commonly used exclusion clause: the obsessions or compulsions are not the result of other mental disorders, such as schizophrenia and related disorders (F20–F29) or mood [affective] disorders (F30–F39) |

# Decision 1: treatment of choice

After diagnosing OCD, the psychiatrist should decide between two first-line therapies: CMI or selective serotonin reuptake inhibitors (SSRIs). Meta-analyses suggesting higher efficacy for less selective agents suffer from methodological limitations, while head-to-head comparisons of CMI and SSRIs have found no difference in efficacy.[8,9] Based on these data, and given that SSRIs are safer and better tolerated, they may be considered the agents of choice. Certainly, if CMI is contraindicated due to a medical condition (such as closed-angle glaucoma, prostatic hypertrophy, or cardiac arrhythmia), then the choice of an SSRI is clear.

Citalopram, fluoxetine, fluvoxamine, paroxetine and sertraline have all been shown effective and well tolerated in randomized

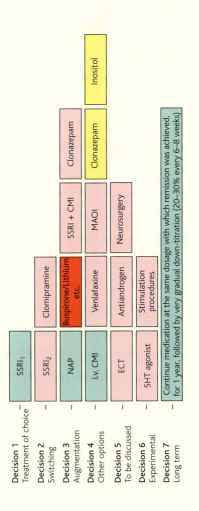

Key
CMI = clomipramine; ECT = electroconvulsive therapy;
i.v. = intravenous formulation; MAOI = monoamine oxidase inhibitor;
NAP = new generation antipsychotic; SSRI₁ = first selective serotonin
reuptake inhibitor*; SSRI₂ = second selective serotonin reuptake inhibitor*

**Figure 7.1** *Treatment decisions for OCD.* ▉ *Intervention supported by consistent randomized trials* ▉ *Intervention supported by limited controlled data* ▉ *Intervention supported by uncontrolled data* ▉ *Interventions that have been found to be ineffective.* (*SSRI₁ denotes treatment of choice; SSRI₂ suggests using a second SSRI after a therapeutic attempt with SSRI₁ has failed.*)

controlled trials of OCD. The few 'head-to-head' comparisons of different SSRIs in OCD show similar efficacy and tolerability.[8]

Fixed-dose studies of OCD are not altogether consistent, but suggest that medication trials in OCD should be of relatively long duration (10–12 weeks) and high dosage (increased to the maximum recommended dose where tolerated).[10] Thus, for example, in the multi-centre citalopram study, there was a trend towards a linear dose–response curve.[11] This recommendation is consistent with a preclinical literature demonstrating that desensitisation of orbitofrontal serotonin receptors is seen only after administration of high doses of SSRIs for significant lengths of time.[12]

## Comorbidity

OCD may be present in a range of different disorders, including psychotic disorders. There is evidence from uncontrolled reports that such cases may benefit from the addition of SSRIs to ongoing antipsychotic treatment.[13]

# Decision 2: switching

If the patient is not able to tolerate adequate doses of SSRIs, or has not responded to an SSRI administered in the upper range of the relevant dose, a different SSRI or CMI may be recommended. There are few empirical data on which to base this choice, although there are data showing that where one SSRI has failed in OCD another may be successful.[14] Given the higher effect size of CMI in OCD meta-analyses,[15,16] some clinicians argue that this medication should be given stronger consideration after failure of one or more SSRI trials.

CMI should be prescribed only in patients without medical contraindications. ECG should be closely monitored, particularly at higher doses, or in patients with concomitant general medical disorders. As in the case of SSRIs, a relatively long trial (10–12 weeks), with high doses where tolerated, is needed. Monitoring of parent drug and desmethyl metabolite levels may be useful in some patients, for example, patients with few side effects may prove to be rapid metabolizers. Caution may be necessary when switching from an SSRI to a TCA, particularly when the SSRI has a long half-life and inhibits cytochrome P450 enzymes.

# Decision 3: augmentation

The question of when to switch and when to augment has received little empirical study in OCD. One approach may, for example, be to switch when there is no response or a partial response to the first trial, to switch or augment if there is a partial response to a second trial, and to augment when there is still no response to a third trial.

Augmentation strategies have focused on decreasing dopamine neurotransmission or further enhancing serotonergic neurotransmission in refractory patients. Indeed, several different agents have been reported to be effective in the augmentation of SRIs.[8] However, in controlled trials, there have been fewer positive findings, with dopamine blockers having the strongest evidence base in support of efficacy.

Early work demonstrated that addition of low doses of traditional antipsychotics was effective, particularly in patients with comorbid tics.[17] Subsequent work has shown that low doses of risperidone, a new generation antipsychotic with a superior side-effect profile, are effective in refractory patients with and without tics.[18] There are also positive studies with other new generation agents.

The data on augmenting agents that potentially enhance serotonergic neurotransmission are less convincing. Controlled trials of buspirone, lithium, inositol and pindolol have either been negative or conflicting.[19,20] Anecdotal reports of fenfluramine and L-tryptophan augmentation have been positive,[21] but fenfluramine is no longer used because of potential cardiac effects, and L-tryptophan has been withdrawn from some markets because of an association with eosinophilia-myalgia syndrome.

There are, however, some controlled data which support the combination of an SSRI with CMI in refractory OCD patients;[22] given the potential of this combination to significantly increase TCA levels, careful monitoring of EEG and drug levels is required.

Clonazepam, a benzodiazepine that may have serotonergic effects, was found effective in a controlled monotherapy study of OCD and in anecdotal reports of augmentation in refractory OCD; it may therefore also be a useful consideration in some patients.[23]

## Decision 4: other options

There is evidence from controlled work that intravenous CMI is effective in refractory OCD. This strategy involves daily infusions of CMI for approximately 14 days, increasing to a maximum dose of 325 mg.[24] Venlafaxine, which has serotonergic effects at lower doses, and both noradrenergic and serotonergic effects at higher doses, may also be useful in some cases of refractory OCD, although further data are needed to support its use.[25]

Early preliminary data suggested that phenelzine might be effective in some OCD patients. However, a placebo-controlled trial of fluoxetine and phenelzine provided no evidence to support the use of phenelzine in OCD.[26] A comparative study of CMI and clorgyline, a reversible inhibitor of monoamine oxidase A, also failed to show any beneficial effect for this agent.[27]

As noted earlier, there are some controlled data supporting the efficacy of clonazepam in OCD. In clinical practice, given the robust effects of the SRIs, use of this agent is typically restricted to augmentation.

An improvement in OCD was reported in one double-blind study of inositol (18 g/day).[28] A replication of these results by another group might help to promote the importance of this novel and essentially safe approach.

## Decision 5: treatments to be discussed

The evidence accumulated so far with regard to the effects of ECT on patients with OCD is in the form of uncontrolled reports and case series.[29] ECT should therefore arguably be reserved for the treatment of severely depressed and suicidal OCD patients.

An early anecdotal report indicated that the antiandrogen cyproterone acetate alleviated OCD symptoms. However, an attempt to replicate this finding by another group failed, and further investigation of antiandrogen therapy is therefore needed.[30]

Neurosurgery may be helpful in patients who remain refractory to a range of other interventions.[31] Current procedures include anterior cingulotomy and anterior capsulotomy. Although well-controlled studies are difficult to perform, several follow-up studies have been published. On the basis of these studies, about 40–60% of patients may receive total or partial benefit from neurosurgery. Some patients who have benefited only partially from neurosurgery may show a better response to previously ineffective treatment modalities. With the advent of new techniques (γ-rays), double-blind sham procedures will be possible, making a controlled study of efficacy possible.

# Decision 6: experimental approaches

Acute administration of specific serotonin agonists, such as mCPP and sumatriptan, has been associated with acute transient exacerbation of OCD symptoms in some patients.[32] Based on the hypothesis that OCD patients are hypersensitive to serotonin agonists, and that the beneficial effect of SSRIs is associated with an adaptive down-regulation of the relevant serotonergic receptors, one may expect that chronic administration of serotonergic agonists will eventually be associated with an improvement of obsessive-compulsive symptoms. Further work is needed to substantiate this idea.

A few case studies have suggested a potential for various novel stimulation techniques (transcranial magnetic stimulation, deep brain stimulation) in the treatment of OCD. However, a controlled study of TMS was negative,[33] and further work is needed to clarify the possible role of such interventions.

# Decision 7: long-term approach

Available data suggest that in most cases the beneficial effects of SSRIs and CMI are maintained as long as the treatments continue. Current clinical consensus indicates that medication should be continued for at least a year after acute treatment response.[10] A number of controlled maintenance studies support this recommendation by demonstrating high rates of relapse after medication discontinuation.[34] Once a decision is made to discontinue medication, a general clinical rule for the anxiety disorders is to taper medication very slowly (for example, decreasing 20–30% of the dose every few months).

# References

1. Wiseman MM, Bland RC, Canino GL, et al. The cross national epidemiology of obsessive-compulsive disorder. *J Clin Psychiatry* 1994; **55**:5–10.
2. Pigott TA, Seay SM. A review of the efficacy of selective serotonin reuptake inhibitors in obsessive-compulsive disorder. *J Clin Psychiatry* 1999; **60**:101–6.
3. Grados MA, Riddle MA. Pharmacological treatment of childhood obsessive-compulsive disorder: from theory to practice. *J Clin Child Psychol* 2001; **30**:67–79.
4. Zohar J, Insel TR. Obsessive compulsive disorder: psychological approaches to diagnosis, treatment and pathophysiology. *Biol Psychiatry* 1987; **22**:667–87.
5. Gross R, Sasson Y, Chopra M, Zohar J. Biological models of obsessive-compulsive disorder. In: Swinson RP, Antony MM, Rachman S, Richter MA, eds. *Obsessive-Compulsive Disorder: Theory, research and treatment*. New York: Guilford Press, 1998:141–53.
6. Abramowitz JS. Effectiveness of psychological and pharmacological treatments for obsessive-compulsive disorder: a quantitative review. *J Consult Clin Psychol* 1997; **65**:44–52.
7. Stein DJ, Fineberg N, Seedat S. An integrated approach to the treatment of OCD. In: Fineberg N, Marazziti D, Stein DJ, eds. *Obsessive-Compulsive Disorder: A practical guide*. London: Martin Dunitz, 2001.
8. Montgomery S, Zohar J. *Obsessive-Compulsive Disorder*. London: Martin Dunitz, 1999.

9.  Zohar J, Sasson Y, Chopra M, et al. Pharmacological treatment of obsessive-compulsive disorder. In: Maj M, Sartorius N, Okasha O, Zohar J, eds. *Obsessive-Compulsive Disorder*. London: John Wiley & Sons, 2000.

10. March JS, Frances A, Carpenter D, et al. Treatment of obsessive-compulsive disorder. The Expert Consensus Panel for obsessive-compulsive disorder. *J Clin Psychiatry* 1997; **58**(Suppl.4):1–72.

11. Montgomery SA, Kasper S, Stein DJ, et al. Citalopram 20mg, 40mg and 60mg are all effective and well tolerated compared with placebo in obsessive compulsive disorder. *Int Clin Psychopharmacol* 2001; **16**:75–86.

12. El Mansari M, Bouchard C, Blier P. Alteration of serotonin release in the guinea pig orbito-frontal cortex by selective serotonin reuptake inhibitors. *Neuropsychopharm* 1995; **13**:117–27.

13. Sasson Y, Bermanzohn P, Zohar J. Treatment of obsessive-compulsive syndromes in schizophrenia. *CNS Spectrums* 1997; **2**:34–45.

14. Marazziti D, Dell'Osso L, Gemignani A, et al. Citalopram in refractory obsessive-compulsive disorder: an open study. *Int Clin Psychopharmacol* 2001; **16**:215–19.

15. Greist J, Jefferson JW, Kobak KA, et al. Efficacy and tolerability of serotonin transport inhibitors in obsessive-compulsive disorder. A meta-analysis. *Arch Gen Psychiatry* 1995; **52**:53–60.

16. Stein D, Spadaccini E, Hollander E. Meta-analysis of pharmacotherapy trials for obsessive compulsive disorder. *Int Clin Psychopharmacol* 1995; **10**:11–18.

17. McDougle CJ, Goodman WK, Leckman JF, et al. Haloperidol addition in fluvoxamine-refractory obsessive-compulsive disorder: a double-blind, placebo-controlled study in patients with and without tics. *Arch Gen Psychiatry* 1994; **51**:302–8.

18. McDougle CJ, Epperson CN, Pelton GH, et al. A double-blind, placebo-controlled study of risperidone addition in serotonin reuptake inhibitor-refractory obsessive-compulsive disorder. *Arch Gen Psychiatry* 2000; **57**:794–802.

19. McDougle CJ, Price LH, Goodman WK, et al. A controlled trial of lithium augmentation in fluvoxamine-refractory obsessive-compulsive disorder: lack of efficacy. *J Clin Psychopharmacol* 1991; **11**:175–81.

20. Grady T, Pigott TA, L'Heureux F, et al. Double-blind study of adjuvant buspirone for fluoxetine-treated patients with obsessive-compulsive disorder. *Am J Psychiatry* 1993; **150**:119–23.

21. Hollander E, DeCaria CM, Schneier F, et al. Fenfluramine augmentation of serotonin reuptake blockade antiobsessional treatment. *J Clin Psychiatry* 1990; **51**:119–23.

22. Ravizza L, Barzega G, Bellino S, et al. Therapeutic effect and safety of adjunctive risperidone in refractory obsessive-compulsive disorder (OCD). *Psychopharmacol Bull* 1996; **32**:677–82.

23. Hewlett WA, Vinogradov S, Agras WS. Clomipramine, clonazepam and clonidine treatment of obsessive-compulsive disorder. *J Clin Psychopharmacol* 1992; **12**:420–30.

24. Koran LM, Sallee FR, Pallanti S. Rapid benefit of intravenous pulse loading of clomipramine in obsessive-compulsive disorder. *Am J Psychiatry* 1997; **154**:396–401.

25. Rauch SL, O'Sullivan RL, Jenike MA. Open treatment of obsessive-compulsive disorder with venlafaxine: a series of ten cases. *J Clin Psychopharmacol* 1996; **16**:81–4.

26. Jenike MA, Baer L, Minichiello WE, et al. Placebo-controlled trial of fluoxetine and phenelzine for obsessive-compulsive disorder. *Am J Psychiatry* 1997; **154**:1261–4.

27. Insel TR, Murphy DL, Cohen RM, Alterman I, Kilts C, Linnoila M. Obsessive-compulsive disorder. A double-blind trial of clomipramine and clorgyline. *Arch Gen Psychiatry* 1984; **40**(6):605–12.

28. Fux M, Levine J, Aviv A, et al. Inositol treatment of obsessive-compulsive disorder. *Am J Psychiatry* 1996; **153**:1219–21.

29. Maletzky B, McFarland B, Burt A. Refractory obsessive compulsive disorder and ECT. *Convuls Ther* 1994; **10**:34–42.

30. Casas M, Alvarez E, Duro P, et al. Antiandrogenic treatment of obsessive-compulsive neurosis. *Acta Psychiatr Scand* 1986; **73**:221–2.

31. Jenike MA. Neurosurgical treatment of obsessive-compulsive disorder. *Br J Psychiatry* 1998; **35**(Suppl.):79–90.

32. Stern L, Zohar J, Hendler T, et al. The potential role of 5-HT1D receptors in the pathophysiology and treatment of obsessive-compulsive disorder. *CNS Spectrums* 1998; **3**:46–9.

33. Alonso P, Pujol J, Cardoner N, et al. Right prefrontal repetitive transcranial magnetic stimulation in obsessive-compulsive disorder: a double-blind, placebo-controlled study. *Am J Psychiatry* 2001; **158**:1143–5.

34. Montgomery SA. Long-term management of obsessive-compulsive disorder. *Int Clin Psychopharmacol* 1997; **11**:23–30.

# Pharmacotherapy of dementia of the Alzheimer's type

## Introduction

Depression and dementia, particularly Alzheimer's disease (AD) and vascular dementia, are the most common psychiatric disorders in the elderly.[1,2] AD accounts for 50–60% of dementia above the age of 60, with prevalence rates doubling every 5 years above the age of 65. This review focuses mainly on AD.

AD is estimated to afflict approximately 13–15 million people worldwide and has been estimated to be the third most costly disease after cancer and heart disease in the USA. It is a progressive neurodegenerative disorder with specific histopathological hallmarks and characteristic clinical features such as progressive impairment of cognition, activities of daily living, behaviour, and quality of life.[1] Molecular and biochemical studies have contributed considerably to the identification of the various steps in its pathogenesis. Symptoms begin in an insidious way, therefore, it is often difficult to date precisely the onset of the disease. Moreover, there is also no specific and reliable early biological marker.[3] Progression is generally gradual. Some 20–50% of patients with AD experience extrapyramidal signs and many suffer from behavioural problems. These additional disorders have been suggested to predict significantly faster cognitive decline.[4]

Many steps are involved in the complex pathogenesis of AD. AD is histopathologically characterized by extracellular deposits of senile plaques composed largely of amyloid b-peptide (Ab) and intracellular deposits of neurofibrillary tangles composed of hyperphosphorylated tau-protein. There is evidence that these cell-damaging events develop 20–30 years before the clinical manifestation of the dementia syndrome. The presence of these histopathological hallmarks correlates clinically with the degree of cognitive dysfunction. Generally, three therapeutic approaches to AD can be differentiated:

- *Slowing symptomatic progression* of the disease, e.g. through new-generation acetylcholinesterase inhibitors with good tolerability and high brain selectivity.
- *Prevention of disease onset*. Various strategies based upon findings, largely from epidemiological research, are under evaluation. These include anti-inflammatories and hormone replacement.
- *Stopping the disease*. This is the major target of compounds (in early stages of development) that aim to modify amyloid and tau-protein metabolism.

In addition to disease-specific treatments, a major target of therapy are the behavioural and psychological symptoms of dementia (BPSD), and reducing BPSD is likely to remain an important goal of treatment even after ever more efficacious disease-modifying and specific treatments.

In order to slow cognitive deterioration, reverse memory deficits and prevent the onset of AD, pharmacotherapy research has focused on six major strategies, as outlined in Table 8.1. These include:

1. Compensation of impaired cholinergic neurotransmission. Of the various attempts, the cholinesterase inhibitors have proved efficacious.
2. Inhibition of the production of neurotoxic free radicals with antioxidants.
3. Promotion of growth of cholinergic neurons with nerve growth factors.
4. Prevention of amyloid deposition and inhibition of the abnormal tau-protein phosphorylation with new compounds.
5. Inhibition of immune and chronic inflammatory mechanisms with anti-inflammatory drugs.

**Table 8.1** Alzheimer's disease — from molecular biology to therapeutics.

| Strategy | Activity | Proposed mechanisms of action | Therapies (examples) |
|---|---|---|---|
| Palliative | Cholinergic mechanisms | Compensation of impaired cholinergic neurotransmission (cholinergic replacement) | Donepezil Rivastigmine Galantamine |
| Neuro-protective | Antagonism of NMDA receptor | Reduction of NMDA activity | Memantine |
| Neuro-protective | Antioxidant | Free-radical scavengers | Vitamin E *Ginkgo biloba* Selegiline |
| Neuro-protective | Neuritic growth | Promotes the growth of cholinergic neurons Interactions with apolipoprotein E Increase of cerebral blood flow and glucose utilization | Oestrogen |
| Neuro-protective | Calcium homeostasis | Reduction of calcium toxicity | Nimodipine |
| Neuro-protective | Anti-inflammatory | Inhibition of immune and chronic inflammatory mechanisms Blockade of microglial activation and cytokine release | Aspirin Indomethacin |
| **Future directions** | | | |
| Prevention | Neuritic growth | Promotion of growth of cholinergic neurons | Nerve growth factor |

*cont.*

*Table 8.1 cont.*

| Prevention | Amyloidogenesis | Modulation of APP gene expression. Prevention of amyloid deposition Degradation of plaques | Protease inhibitors Anti-fibrillation therapy 'Amyloid vaccine' |
|---|---|---|---|
| Prevention | Tau-processing | Inhibition of phosphorylation of tau-protein. Prevention of tau aggregation | Kinase inhibitors Anti-fibrillation therapy |

The role of general practitioners and psychiatrists has changed considerably with the introduction of new and effective treatments. It is likely, but remains to be satisfactorily proven, that early intervention leads to a delay in institutionalization and to an improvement in quality of life for patients and caregivers. The intensive cooperation between physicians, psychiatrists, patients and their families is essential for adequate treatment. It is important to inform the caregivers about the diagnosis, the possible causes of the disease, its prognosis and the available treatments as well as basic strategies of care. Increasingly, many clinicians also discuss the diagnosis with the patient, a change in practice mirroring that within oncology a decade or two previously. Discussing diagnosis with the patient is often difficult and can be painful for the patient, the carer and, indeed, the clinician. However, with the drive towards ever earlier diagnosis, patients will increasingly present while having sufficient cognitive ability to understand the diagnosis and to plan for the future. It is also important to advise patients and caregivers on the available sources of care, financial and legal issues that may arise, and the risk of accidents due to impaired cognitive performance. Different programmes have been developed for relieving the stress and frustration or depression of caregivers.

The treatment strategy depends on the severity of the illness. Recent studies have demonstrated that non-cognitive symptoms such as irritability, aggression and sleep disturbances are the most distressing for caregivers. Carers may not realize that these symptoms are part of the disease process. There is some evidence that behavioural disturbances correlate with the different stages of cognitive deterioration associated with AD. Behavioural symptoms seem to be more common during moderate stages. In severe stages, significant cognitive impairment is predominant and behavioural disturbances less problematic. However, this may be because some BPSD are harder to detect in the later stages. The patient may be as depressed as before but the only 'symptom' is decreased activity and anorexia, rather than crying and observable diurnal variation in mood. Some behaviours, such as distressing abnormal vocalizations, become more common as the disease progresses. Characteristic features in the early stages are impairment of memory for recent events and mild loss of intellectual abilities. Clinical 'steps' in the pharmacotherapy of dementia of the Alzheimer's type (DAT) therefore include:

1. Establishment of a diagnosis.
2. Development of a treatment plan.
3. Pharmacological treatment of cognitive dysfunction.
4. Diagnosis and pharmacotherapy of behavioural disturbances in dementia.

## Step 1: diagnosis of a dementia syndrome

The diagnosis of a dementia syndrome is established by clinical history, physical examination and neuropsychological tests, supplemented by biochemical analysis, with brain imaging necessary in some, but not all cases. Referral to a specialist may be required in early diagnosis, particularly when differentiating benign, age-related cognitive changes from mild cognitive impairment and the early stages of AD. Specialist consultation may also be helpful in severe cases as well as those with behavioural disturbances and other comorbid conditions.

ICD-10 and DSM-IV (Table 8.2) provide clinical diagnostic criteria for AD and other forms of dementia. More specialized criteria for the sub-types of the common forms of dementia, including AD,[5] vascular dementia,[6] dementia with Lewy bodies (DLB)[7] and fronto-temporal dementia[8] have been published. Using the NINCDS-ADRDA criteria for AD, three levels of certainty in diagnosis are recognized:

- possible AD, where the clinical picture is atypical or there is some other confounding disease process;
- probable AD, with a typical slowly progressive decline;
- definite AD, a post-mortem-confirmed diagnosis.

The clinical diagnosis of probable AD is confirmed in approximately 80–90% cases by autopsy. The diagnostic process involves three steps:

- identifying cognitive loss or 'confusion';
- determining that there is a dementia syndrome and its differentiation from normal ageing, mild cognitive impairment and delirium;
- finally, the nosological differentiation (AD, DLB, dementia of frontal lobe type, Parkinson's disease, Huntington's disease or cerebrovascular disease).

The exclusion of reversible or potentially curable causes of dementia is crucial. These include vitamin $B_{12}$ deficiency, endocrine and metabolic dysfunctions, infections, space-occupying lesions, and normal pressure hydrocephalus.

The first step in this process is one of the most important. Much dementia is unrecognized – only approximately 60% of those with dementia were correctly identified by general practitioners in one study, for example.[9] This was conducted in an area known to have a comprehensive and highly developed primary care network. A major goal of dementia services worldwide is to improve detection rates of dementia. One important approach to this is the use of screening instruments in primary care – scales such as the Abbreviated Mental Test score and the Clock Drawing Test are

*Table 8.2* *Diagnostic criteria for dementia of the Alzheimer's type.*

## DSM-IV criteria for dementia of the Alzheimer type (code 290.xx)

A. The development of multiple cognitive deficits manifested by both:
- memory impairment (impaired ability to learn new information and to recall previously learned information)
- one (or more) of the following cognitive disturbances:
  aphasia
  apraxia
  agnosia
  disturbance in executive functioning

B. The cognitive deficits in criteria cause significant impairment in social or occupational functioning

C. Characteristic gradual onset and continuing cognitive decline

D. The cognitive deficits in criteria A are not caused by:
- other central nervous system conditions causing progressive deficits in memory and cognition (e.g. cerebrovascular disease, Parkinson's disease, Huntington's disease, subdural haematoma, normal pressure hydrocephalus, brain tumour)
- systemic conditions known to cause dementia (e.g. hypothyroidism, vitamin $B_{12}$ or folic acid deficiency, niacin deficiency, hypercalcaemia, neurosyphilis, HIV infection)
- substance-induced conditions

E. The deficits do not occur exclusively during the course of a delirium

F. Symptoms not better accounted for by another Axis I disorder (e.g. major depressive disorder, schizophrenia)

Note: Code is based on type of onset and predominant features. Also code Alzheimer's disease on Axis III

## ICD-10 criteria for dementia of the Alzheimer type (category F00)

A. The general criteria for dementia (G1–G4) must be met

B. Diagnosis of dementia:
- memory impairment (new information)
- cognitive disturbances (language, executive function, agnosia, apraxia)
- significant impairment in social and/or occupational functioning, decline from previous level
- duration of at least 6 months

*cont.*

*Table 8.2* cont.

| C. Gradual onset and continuing decline |
| --- |
| D. There is no evidence from the history, physical examination or special investigations for any other possible cause of dementia (e.g. cerebrovascular disease, HIV disease, Parkinson's disease, Huntington's disease, normal pressure hydrocephalus), a systemic disorder (e.g. hypothyroidism, vitamin $B_{12}$ or folic acid deficiency, hypercalcaemia), or alcohol or drug abuse |

Characteristic features of DLB are fluctuating cognition, recurrent visual hallucinations, disturbances of vigilance, delusions, parkinsonism, falls and neuroleptic hypersensitivity.

rapid screens suitable for use in primary care, particularly if supplemented by more comprehensive measures, such as the Mini Mental State Examination (MMSE).[10] Having determined the presence of cognitive impairment, the next task is vital to rapidly distinguish this from delirium. Again, this is a primary-care process based upon assessment of consciousness, physical examination and a good history from an informant.

The specific diagnosis is important and increasingly the use of relatively standardized criteria for the different dementias is leading to improved accuracy. Examples of clinical decisions that might flow from accurate differential diagnosis include the avoidance of neuroleptics in DLB if at all possible, consideration of aspirin and optimizing hypertension treatment in those with vascular dementia, and the use of cholinesterase inhibitors in AD.

# Step 2: development of a management plan

After diagnosing a dementia syndrome, the clinician should develop a management plan including family interventions, treatment of cognitive dysfunctions, therapy of associated somatic diseases and mood and behavioural management. This starts with discussion of the diagnosis and prognosis with carers, with family members, and increasingly with patients where this is considered appropriate. Lay societies are an important resource and offer much support and families often benefit from having alternative sources of information. Alzheimer's Disease International is the umbrella group for national societies and helps to initiate and support national societies where they are not well developed (http://www.alz.co.uk/).

Formulation of a management plan will be specific to the individual and will need to be regularly reviewed. Ideally, a management plan will be constructed by a multidisciplinary team as the programme may have input from the general practitioner, the specialist (if a neurologist, then psychiatrists should also be involved to manage BPSD), community nurses, social services, voluntary services, psychology and occupational therapy. Rarely is such an ideal met, but the clinician should call upon other disciplines to ensure a comprehensive care package. Elements of the management plan are outlined in Figures 8.1 and 8.2.

# Step 3: pharmacological treatment of cognitive dysfunction

Acetylcholinesterase (AChE) inhibitors were the first compounds to be approved for Alzheimer's disease.

## First- and second-generation acetylcholinesterase inhibitors

Multiple neurotransmitter deficits occur in AD, including dopaminergic, noradrenergic and serotonergic systems. However, the most significant degeneration occurs in cholinergic pathways, which are most directly linked to cognitive function. Thus, restoration of cholinergic neurotransmission may be most important for ameliorating impaired memory and learning. Indeed, a direct correlation has been demonstrated between cholinesterase (ChE) inhibition and cognitive performance.

The efficacy of AChE inhibitors is dependent on the functioning of the presynaptic neuron releasing acetylcholine. With the progression of the disease, and the resulting degeneration of cholinergic neurons, it would be predicted that the clinical efficacy of AChE inhibitors would be reduced. However, it remains to be proven at

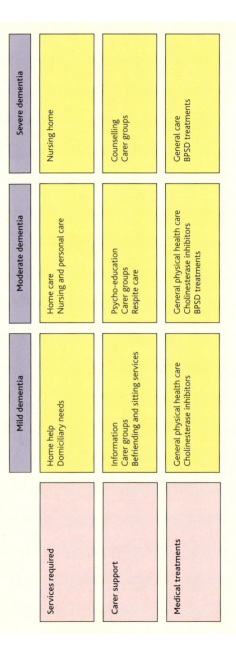

*Figure 8.1* Management issues change as the disease progresses.

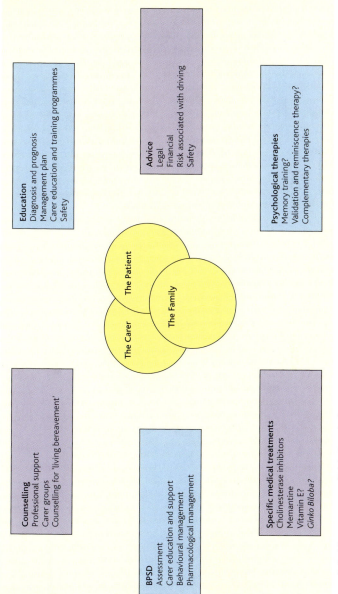

**Counselling**
Professional support
Carer groups
Counselling for 'living bereavement'

**Education**
Diagnosis and prognosis
Management plan
Carer education and training programmes
Safety

**Advice**
Legal
Financial
Risk associated with driving
Safety

The Patient

The Carer

The Family

**BPSD**
Assessment
Carer education and support
Behavioural management
Pharmacological management

**Specific medical treatments**
Cholinesterase inhibitors
Memantine
Vitamin E?
*Ginko Biloba?*

**Psychological therapies**
Memory training?
Validation and reminiscence therapy?
Complementary therapies

*Figure 8.2* *Management of Alzheimer's disease*

91

what stage in the disease this occurs. These compounds have been demonstrated to slow the symptomatic progression of the disease significantly over months or years, thus improving the quality of life of patients and caregivers and possibly delaying nursing home placement. It is possible that replacing the declining cholinergic function would have a disease-modifying effect by reducing amyloidogenic metabolism and reducing tau-phosphorylation.[11] This has yet to be demonstrated in patients but might underlie the otherwise puzzling observation that delayed treatment is less efficacious.

**Tacrine** and **physostigmine** were first-generation cholinesterase inhibitors. The efficacy of tacrine in the therapy of mild-to-moderate AD was demonstrated in a number of double-blind, placebo-controlled trials. Moreover, it has been found that tacrine, in higher doses, is capable of delaying nursing home placement.[12] However, low oral bioavailability, gastrointestinal side effects and hepatic toxicity limited the use of this compound. High potential for liver toxicity requires continuous monitoring of serum transaminase levels during treatment and tacrine can no longer be considered as a first-line treatment in patients with AD.

**Donepezil** is a piperidine-based reversible AChE inhibitor with a half-life of approximately 70 hours. Excellent tolerability and safety profiles, as well as clinical efficacy in short- and long-term use, in doses up to 10 mg/day, have been demonstrated in a number of placebo-controlled trials of patients with mild-to-moderate AD.[13] Treatment recommendations are for a starting dose of 5 mg/day in a single evening dose; with dose increased on the basis of tolerability to 10 mg/day after 4–6 weeks. As with other AChE inhibitors, gastrointestinal side effects, agitation, dizziness and insomnia may be observed. These side effects are often mild, transient and resolve without dose modification.

**Rivastigmine**, a pseudo-irreversible AChE inhibitor of the carbamate type, has an elimination half-life of 2 hours but as it is a pseudo-irreversible inhibitor, it has a pharmacological half-life of approximately 12 hours.[14] Its clinical profile may be comparable with donepezil although rivastigmine also inhibits butyrylcholinesterase. Treatment recommendations are for a starting dose of 1.5 mg twice daily; with dose increased up to 3 mg twice daily after 2–3 weeks, to a maximum dosage of 6 mg twice daily. Clinical trials demonstrated a dose–response relationship with the lower doses being ineffective. In certain patients, one or more of the following side effects may occur: nausea and vomiting, anorexia, weight loss, peptic ulcers/gastro-intestinal bleeding, exaggerated muscle relaxation during anaesthesia, and cardiovascular, genitourinary, neurological and pulmonary conditions.

**Galantamine** is the most recently licensed compound in this class and has demonstrated comparable efficacy to other AChE inhibitors as well as tolerability/safety in AD patients.[15] The half-life is 7 hours and the treatment recommendations comprise a twice-daily regime of between 4 mg and 12 mg. In addition to cholinesterase inhibition, galantamine binds to the nicotinic receptor enhancing pre-synaptic acetylcholine release – so called allosteric modulation. It remains to be seen whether this pharmacological effect has any clinical consequences.

In summary, compared with tacrine, which can be viewed as a first-generation AChE inhibitor, the clinical efficacy and in particular the safety and tolerability of second-generation AChE inhibitors, such as donepezil, galantamine and rivastigmine, are generally better.[16] The incidence of peripheral cholinergic side effects is low and typically of mild intensity, as the compounds are highly specific for brain acetylcholinesterase and, compared with tacrine, longer-lasting.

A number of clinical decisions present themselves to the clinician considering prescribing one of these compounds:

1. when to start
2. when to stop
3. how to monitor
4. how to choose
5. what to tell relatives.

## When to start
These compounds were assessed first for efficacy in mild-to-moderate Alzheimer's disease. All patients fitting this category should

therefore be considered for treatment, and the first guidelines to be published suggested possible or probable AD with MMSE scores between 10 and 24 to be suitable.[17] As data accumulate showing that the compounds may also be efficacious (possibly even more so) in other dementias (for example, DLB), the criteria for treatment will need to be reconsidered. Other data also suggest that the cholinesterase inhibitors have efficacy in treating the behavioural symptoms in dementia, and some have suggested that this class of drugs are effectively a new class of psychotropics.[18] In summary, then, the cholinesterase inhibitors should be started as early as practicable in those with mild or moderate AD, and consideration should be given to those with DLB and to those with AD plus BPSD.

**When to stop**

All drugs have side effects, and few work indefinitely. This class of treatment is no exception and consideration should be given to stopping treatment when the drug is having no effect. Determining this point is difficult. Two types of treatment failure can be distinguished – primary failure or non-response, and, secondary failure or those who do respond but then lose response. Primary failure is relatively straightforward to observe but not possible to predict. A proportion (the exact percentage is not clear and depends upon definition) of patients continue to deteriorate after starting the drug at the same rate as before. Sequential cognitive testing is rarely available in a clinical setting, and so determination of primary failure is achieved largely through informant interview. It is probably not possible to determine primary failure before 3 months and some would continue treatment for 6 months. If after this time the patient has continued to deteriorate noticeably to the informant, then this can be taken as clinical primary failure. Secondary treatment failure is harder to determine. If the patient shows little or no deterioration for a period longer than 6 months and then begins to deteriorate again, it is possible that the drug has ceased to work, but equally plausible that deterioration would be even faster without treatment. In this situation a 'drug holiday' can help. If after stopping the drug deterioration accelerates, then it can be concluded that there was some efficacy and the drug can be re-instated. In summary, then, cholinesterase inhibitors should be given for 3–6 months' minimum to determine efficacy. 'Drug holidays' can help to decide if deterioration is due to secondary treatment failure.

## How to monitor

Primary and secondary failure can be assessed only by careful monitoring. Efficacy has been demonstrated in clinical trials in the domains of cognition, function and behaviour. Monitoring should therefore assess each of these domains. A good clinical assessment and informant interview are essential but they can be supplemented by appropriate scales. Choice of scales is a matter of judgement but a compromise is inevitably necessary between practicability and scientific rigour. Rarely are the robust assessment procedures necessary in clinical trials practicable in clinical practice. A package of assessment procedures might include an MMSE, a Bristol Activity of Daily Living scale, a neuropsychiatric inventory and a CIBIC-plus.[10] This might be supplemented by a FAST staging and a relative stress scale. Such a package can be completed in approximately 30 minutes and is therefore suitable for use in most routine clinical practices.

## How to choose

At present, the clinician is frustrated in attempting to make an evidence-based choice between compounds. In order to assess relative efficacy suitably large and prolonged head-to-head comparisons will be necessary. Attempting to distinguish between compounds on the basis of the relative treatment–placebo differences is to be avoided, as careful scrutiny demonstrates that the most pronounced difference between the various published trials is the rate of deterioration of the placebo group. Other factors therefore come into play. Given no obvious and apparent differences in efficacy, drug costs will be considered important in many cases. Ease of use is of primary importance – donepezil has the longest half-life and can be given as a once-daily regimen. This is a distinct advantage over the other compounds where a patient is taking no other medication. Where the patient already has multiple daily supervised medication, the advantage is less apparent. The relative side effects can be determined readily from single compound clinical trials.[19–21]

In summary, no good head-to-head trial has yet been published to determine relative efficacy. Choosing between compounds therefore involves consideration of tolerability, costs and ease of use.

**What to tell relatives**
Managing expectations is all-important in treating dementia. These compounds are modestly efficacious and can be expected to slow down the rate of deterioration of symptoms. Until proven otherwise, it must be assumed that the disease process will continue unabated, and relatives should be informed of this. Involving relatives early will help to avert the devastation and sense of hopelessness otherwise engendered in some when the clinician decides the time has come to stop treatment. Appropriately forewarned, most relatives accept this process and are able to move on. Managing expectations is also important when it comes to those paying for health care. As long as treatment is restricted to those with mild or moderate, largely incident (as opposed to prevalent) disease, the numbers needing treatment are relatively modest.

## Antioxidants

The production of neurotoxic free radicals by the ageing process itself, and in particular by the β-amyloid protein, has been suggested to be one of the major mechanisms of neurodegeneration in dementia syndromes.[22–24] The accumulation of free radicals causes oxidative stress leading to lipid peroxidation in the membranes and neuronal degeneration. Antioxidants, such as vitamin E and selegeline, have been suggested to improve cognitive impairment.[25] Other study results suggest that β-carotene, vitamin E or glutathione improve immune function in the elderly.

In a large double-blind, placebo-controlled multicentre trial, 341 patients with AD of moderate severity received either the selective monoamine oxidase-B (MAO-B) inhibitor, selegeline (10 mg/day), or the α-tocopherol, vitamin E (2000 IU/day), or both selegeline and vitamin E, or placebo, for 2 years.[25] It was found that treatment with selegeline or α-tocopherol, and the combination of both compounds, significantly slowed the progression of the disease compared with placebo, delaying the deterioration of the performance of activities of daily living. Both selegeline and vitamin E were well tolerated. Vitamin E should be dosed at 400–800 IU/day. (Doses between 200 and 2000 IU/day have been shown to be well tolerated. However, there are no conclusive dose–relationship studies available to date.) Selegeline should be dosed at 5–10 mg/day. Orthostatic hypotension, agitation, hypertensive crises and adverse drug interactions are possible side effects. Vitamin E has been suggested to be preferable to selegeline in the APA guidelines because it is less expensive, has a more favourable side-effect profile and less potential for medication interactions. However, whether either compound can be recommended as a result of this single trial is questioned by many.

## Anti-inflammatory drugs

There is some evidence to suggest that involvement of the immune system and inflammatory mechanisms may be important in the pathogenesis of AD. Specifically, the risk of AD or disease progression has been suggested to be diminished among those with a prior history of treatment with anti-inflammatory drugs (indomethacin, prednisone).[26–28] However, these findings are primarily based on retrospective analysis, and results from prospective trials are pending.

## Oestrogen replacement therapy

There is some evidence that the oestrogen loss associated with menopause may contribute to the development of AD.[29] Oestrogen has multiple functions in the CNS, including stimulation of neuritic growth, synapse formation, promotion of the amyloid precursor protein to fragments less likely to aggregate than β-amyloid, modification of inflammatory responses, antioxidant properties, improving regional cerebral blood flow, increasing cerebral blood glucose utilization and activating the cholinergic system. There is some evidence to suggest that oestrogen use in postmenopausal women may delay the onset and decrease the risk of AD. These findings support the hypothesis of a protective influence of oestrogen in AD. However, since available prospective data are presently limited, no conclusive recommendations can be made at the present time. The decision to initiate oestrogen replacement therapy should be made together with a gynaecologist weighing the risks and benefits of this approach.

## Memantine

Memantine is an NMDA receptor antagonist already widely pre-scribed in some European countries.[30] Emerging data suggest that this compound might be efficacious for AD, especially in the severe stages.[31,32]

## Others

A particular extract of *Ginkgo biloba* (EGb 761) is used in Europe to treat cognitive dysfunction. The EGb extract contains multiple compounds that are thought to act synergistically on diverse processes involved in the homeostasis of inflammation and oxida-tive stress. Its main effect seems to be related to antioxidant and anti-inflammatory properties, thus inhibiting lipid peroxidation and cell damage. In a controlled trial,[33] a small but statistically signifi-cant drug–placebo group difference was found in patients with AD and multi-infarct dementia. EGb was well tolerated and therefore used in a large number of sub-threshold cases. The recommended dosage is 40 mg three times daily. Interactions with other medica-tions need to be taken into account. Further studies are necessary, in particular to clarify the dose–response relationship and clinical efficacy compared with AChE inhibitors. *Other nootropics*, such as piracetam, nimodipine and co-dergocrine mesylate, have been reported to improve some neuropsychological and behavioural parameters in patients with specific and non-specific cognitive impairment.

## Treatment decision for the pharmacotherapy of AD

Treatment strategies are based on the knowledge that various bio-logical mechanisms are involved in the pathogenesis of AD, including amyloid pathogenesis, the neurotoxicity of free radicals, abnormal phosphorylation and the large number of neurotransmit-ter deficits.

Figure 8.3 summarizes possible treatment strategies targeting dif-ferent crucial steps in the pathogenesis of AD. At present there are no large controlled trials available for one or the other augmenta-tion treatment strategy; this needs to be substantiated in further studies.

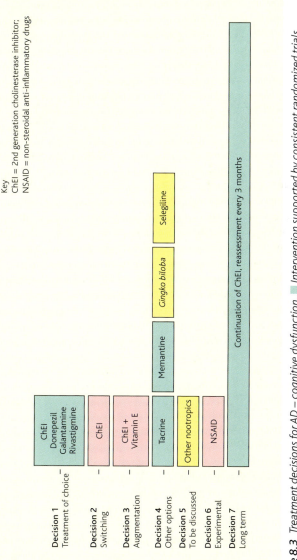

**Figure 8.3** Treatment decisions for AD – cognitive dysfunction. ■ Intervention supported by consistent randomized trials ■ Intervention supported by limited controlled data ■ Intervention supported by uncontrolled data.

Key
ChEI = 2nd generation cholinesterase inhibitor;
NSAID = non-steroidal anti-inflammatory drugs

**Decision 1**
Treatment of choice – ChEI
Donepezil
Galantamine
Rivastigmine

**Decision 2**
Switching – ChEI

**Decision 3**
Augmentation – ChEI +
Vitamin E

**Decision 4**
Other options – Tacrine | Memantine | Gingko biloba | Selegiline

**Decision 5**
To be discussed – Other nootropics

**Decision 6**
Experimental – NSAID

**Decision 7**
Long term – Continuation of ChEI, reassessment every 3 months

# Step 4: diagnosis and pharmacotherapy of behavioural disturbances in dementia

Behavioural disturbances are common and important features of dementia (see Table 8.2) and more prominent in moderate stages.[34] This is not surprising when AD involves multiple degeneration implicating the cholinergic system, serotonin and noradrenaline. For example, alterations in serotonergic neurotransmission may be associated with either depression or psychosis depending on the functional integrity of other neurotransmitter systems. Neurodegenerative processes in various brain regions, including neurotransmitter imbalances, constitute the physiological substrate, whereas personality and psychological factors play a modifying role.

Depressive symptoms occur in 20–60% of patients in AD and 10–30% meet criteria for major depressive episode. There is some evidence that the newer generation of antidepressants, in particular the SSRIs (e.g. citalopram 20 mg/day, paroxetine 20 mg/day and sertraline 50 mg/day), may exert beneficial effects on cognition and behavioural disturbances in addition to the well-known antidepressive properties. Traditional tricyclic antidepressants should be avoided, if possible, due to significant anticholinergic side effects.

## Anxiety

Anxiety occurs in 50–80% of patients with AD, often together with depressive symptomatology. Antidepressant medications, particularly SSRIs, are likely to improve both syndromes. Benzodiazepines should be used with caution in demented patients with anxiety because of the risk of worsening cognitive function (via sedation), delirium and the risk of gait disturbances. If used, short-acting compounds without active metabolites, such as lorazepam (0.5–1 mg every 4–6 hours) and oxazepam, are recommended. Note that benzodiazepine dependence is not a primary problem in AD.

## Delusions and hallucinations

Psychotic symptoms are frequent (40–80% of AD patients) and prominent manifestations of AD, particularly in the moderate and severe stages. Delusions appear to be more frequent than hallucinations. Most patients benefit from low doses of the new generation antipsychotics, with a significantly lower potential for extrapyramidal side effects (e.g. olanzapine, quetiapine, risperidone, sertindole and ziprasidone).[4] However, to date, clinical data on the use of these new compounds (with the exception of risperidone) in dementia are limited. Patients with DLB are highly sensitive to antipsychotics and should be treated only with atypical compounds (e.g. clozapine in low doses such as 25 mg) with low extrapyramidal side effects.[35]

## Aggression

Aggressive behaviour is one of the most challenging behavioural disturbances in dementia, occurring in up to 60% of all patients. Low-potency antipsychotics with a low anticholinergic potential may be helpful (e.g. pipamperone 20–120 mg/day, risperidone 0.5–2 mg/day) or alternatively benzodiazepines or SSRIs.

## Agitation and wandering

Agitation and wandering in dementia increase with the duration and severity of the illness. Numerous, non-pharmacological treatment approaches have been described, including behavioural management, environmental modifications, including sound and light, and social interaction groups. Low doses of new generation neuroleptics, benzodiazepines and SSRIs may be helpful.

## Sleep disturbances

Sleep disturbances in AD are characterized by fragmented sleep or interruption in the day–night sleep cycling. Low-potency antipsychotics with low anticholinergic effects (e.g. pipamperone 10–60 mg/day), and new non-benzodiazepine hypnotics, such as zolpidem (10 mg/day) and zopiclone (3.75–7.5 mg/day), may be particularly useful.

# Summary and long-term treatment perspective

Depression and dementia are the most common psychiatric disorders in the elderly. AD accounts for 50–60% of dementia above the age of 60. Intensive co-operation between general physicians, primary care physicians, psychiatrists, patients and their families is essential for the adequate management of these illnesses. After diagnosis of dementia, a treatment plan should be developed, including family interventions, treatment of cognitive dysfunction, therapy of associated somatic diseases and mood and behavioural management. Early diagnosis and therapy of reversible or potentially curable causes of dementia is of utmost importance.[36]

Second-generation AChE inhibitors have been found to improve cognitive dysfunction in patients with mild-to-moderate AD and are currently the drugs of choice. These new compounds are highly specific for brain AChE and generally well tolerated. In addition, they may have beneficial effects on behavioural disorders. The initial treatment duration should be at least 6–12 months, the response should be reassessed at 3–6 monthly intervals in order to decide if switching or augmentation is indicated. Side effects may necessitate intervention before 3 months. Antioxidants, such as vitamin E and selegeline, and anti-inflammatory drugs, as well as oestrogen replacement therapy, may have positive effects on the disease process. They have been suggested as second-line agents.

AD is a complex disorder and many steps are involved in its pathogenesis, which may require combination treatment strategies. Behavioural disturbances such as irritability, aggression and sleep disturbances are the most distressing symptoms for caregivers and require a different pharmacological treatment approach to that used for cognitive symptoms.

## References

1. American Psychiatric Association. Practice guideline for the treatment of patients with Alzheimer's disease and other dementias of late life. *Am J Psychiatry* 1997; **154**(Suppl.5):1–39.
2. Bancher C, Croy A, Dal Bianco P, et al. Österreichisches Alzheimer-Krankheit-Konsensuspapier. *Neuropsychiatrie* 1998; **3**:126–67.
3. Ritchie K, Kildea D. Is senile dementia 'age-related' or 'ageing-related'? Evidence from meta-analysis of dementia prevalence in the oldest old. *Lancet* 1995; **346**:931–4.

4. Chui HC, Lyness SA, Sobel E, et al. Extrapyramidal signs and psychiatric symptoms predict faster cognitive decline in Alzheimer's disease. *Arch Neurol* 1994; **51**:676–81.

5. McKhann G, Drachman D, Folstein M, et al. Clinical diagnosis of Alzheimer's disease: report of the NINCDS-ADRDA Work Group under the auspices of Department of Health and Human Services Task Force on Alzheimer's Disease. *Neurology* 1984; **34**:939–44.

6. Roman GC, Tatemichi TK, Erkinjuntti T, et al. Vascular dementia: diagnostic criteria for research studies. Report of the NINDS-AIREN International Workshop. *Neurology* 1993; **43**(2):250–60.

7. McKeith IG, Galasko D, Kosaka K, et al. Consensus guidelines for the clinical and pathologic diagnosis of dementia with Lewy bodies (DLB): Report of the consortium on DLB international workshop. *Neurology* 1996; **47**:1113–24.

8. Neary D, Snowden JS, Gustafson L, et al. Frontotemporal lobar degeneration: a consensus on clinical diagnostic criteria. *Neurology* 1998; **51**(6):1546–54.

9. O'Connor DW, Pollitt PA, Hyde JB, et al. Do general practitioners miss dementia in elderly patients? *BMJ* 1988; **297**:1107–10.

10. Burns A, Lawlor B, Craig S. *Assessment Scales in Old Age Psychiatry*. London: Martin Dunitz, 1999.

11. Francis PT, Palmer AM, Snape M, Wilcock GK. The cholinergic hypothesis of Alzheimer's disease: a review of progress. *J Neurol Neurosurg Psychiatry* 1999; **66**:137–47.

12. Knopman D, Schneider L, Davis K, et al. Long-term tacrine (Cognex) treatment: effects on nursing home placement and mortality. Tacrine Study Group. *Neurology* 1996; **47**:166–77.

13. Rogers SL, Friedhoff LT. Long-term efficacy and safety of donepezil in the treatment of Alzheimer's disease: an interim analysis of the results of a US multicentre open label extension study. *Euro Neuropsychopharm* 1997; **8**:67–75.

14. Anand R, Hartmann R, Hayes P. An overview of the development of SDZ ENA 713, a brain selective cholinesterase inhibitor. In: Becker R, Giacobini E, eds. *Alzheimer Disease: From molecular biology to therapy*. Boston: Birkhäuser, 1996:239–43.

15. Rainer ML, Mucke HAM. Twenty years of cholinergic intervention in Alzheimer's disease: a tale of disappointment and ultimate confidence. *Int J Psychiatry Clin Prac* 1998; **2**:173–9.

16. Giacobini E. Cholinesterase inhibitors for Alzheimer's disease therapy: from tacrine to future applications. *Neurochem Int*. 1998; **32**:413–19.

17. Lovestone S, Graham N, Howard R. Guidelines on drug treatments for Alzheimer's disease. *Lancet* 1997; **350**:232–3.

18. Cummings JL, Donohue JA, Brooks RL. The relationship between donepezil and behavioral disturbances in patients with Alzheimer's disease. *Am J Geriatr Psychiatry* 2000; **8**:134–40.

19. Rogers SL, Friedhoff LT. Long-term efficacy and safety of donepezil in the treatment of Alzheimer's disease: an interim analysis of the results of a US multicentre open label extension study. *Eur Neuropsychopharmacol* 1998; **8**:67–75.

20. Birks J, Iakovidou V, Tsolaki M. Rivastigmine for Alzheimer's disease. *Cochrane Database Syst Rev*, 2000.

21. Tariot PN, Solomon PR, Morris JC, et al. A 5-month, randomized, placebo-controlled trial of galantamine in AD. *Neurology* 2000; **54**:2269–76.

22. Meydani S, Wu D, Santos S. Antioxidants and immune response in aged persons: overview of present evidence. *Am J Clin Nutr* 1995; **62**(Suppl):1462–76.

23. Behl C. Alzheimer's disease and oxidative stress: implications for novel therapeutic approaches. *Progr Neurobiol* 1999; **57**:301–23.

24. Pitchumoni SS, Doraiswamy PM. Current status of antioxidant therapy for Alzheimer's disease. *J Am Geriatr Soc* 1998; **46**:1566–72.

25. Sano M, Ernesto C, Thomas RG, et al. A controlled trial of selegiline, alpha-tocopherol, or both as treatment for Alzheimer's disease. *N Engl J Med* 1997; **336**:1216–22.

26. Aisen P, Davis K. Inflammatory mechanisms in Alzheimer's disease: implications for therapy. *Am J Psychiatry* 1994; **151**:1105–13.

27. Breitner JCS. Inflammatory processes and anti-inflammatory drugs in Alzheimer's disease: a current appraisal. *Neurobiol of Ageing* 1996; **17**:5789–94.

28. Stewart WF, Kawas C, Corrada M, et al. Risk of Alzheimer's disease and duration of NSAID use. *Neurology* 1997; **48**:626–32.

29. Paganini-Hill A, Henderson VW. Oestrogen replacement therapy and risk of Alzheimer disease. *Arch Intern Med* 1996; **156**:2213–17.

30. Förstl H. Clinical issues in current drug therapy for dementia. *Alzheimer Dis Assoc Disord* 2000; **14**(Suppl.1):S103–8.

31. Marx J. Alzheimer's congress. Drug shows promise for advanced disease. *Science* 2000; **289**:375–7.

32. Winblad B, Poritis N. Memantine in severe dementia: results of the 9M-Best Study (Benefit and efficacy in severely demented patients during treatment with memantine). *Int J Geriatr Psychiatry*

**14**:135–46.
33. Le Bars PLC, Katz MM, Berman N, et al. A placebo-controlled, double-blind randomised trial of an extract of Ginkgo biloba for dementia. *JAMA* 1997; **278**:1327–32.
34. Müller-Spahn F, Hock C. Behavioural disturbances in old age. In: Lader M, Naber D, eds. *Difficult Clinical Problems in Psychiatry*. London: Martin Dunitz, 1999:181–98.
35. McKeith I, Galasko D, Kosaka K, et al. Clinical and pathological diagnosis of dementia with Lewy bodies (DLB): report of the CDLB international workshop. *Neurology* 1996; **47**:1113–24.
36. Small GW, Rabins PV, Barry PP, et al. Diagnosis and treatment of Alzheimer's disease and related disorders. Consensus statement of the American Association for Geriatric Psychiatry, the Alzheimer's Association, and the American Geriatrics Society. *JAMA* 1997; **278**:1363–71.

# Index

Numbers in italics indicate *tables* or *figures*.

acetylcholinesterase (AChE)
        inhibitors in AD
    choice of drug 95
    drugs 91–2
    efficacy 91
    managing expectations of
        treatment 95–6
    monitoring treatment 95
    starting treatment 93
    stopping treatment 94
    treatment failure 94
AD *see* Alzheimer's disease
        (AD)
aggression in dementia 101
agitation in dementia 101
alprazolam 42
Alzheimer's disease (AD)
        81–105
    behavioural and psychological
        symptoms (BPSD) 82,
        84–5, 100–1
    cooperation in patient care 84
    diagnosis 85–8, *87–8*
    long-term treatment 102
    management plan 88–91, *90,
        91*
    pathogenesis 81–2
    prevalence 81
    strategies in pharmacotherapy
        research 82, *83*
    therapeutic approaches 82
    treatment of behavioural
        disturbances 98, 100–1
    treatment of cognitive
        dysfunction 89–99, *99*
Alzheimer's Disease
        International 88
amitriptyline 64
antidepressants
    bipolar depression 15, 16, 19
    comorbid disorders in
        schizophrenia 30
    depressive symptoms in AD
        100
    dual 4
    intravenous 7, 18
    OCD 69, 71, 72–4
    panic disorder 38–9, 41, 43
    PTSD 62, 64
    social anxiety 51, 52–3, 54
    unipolar depression 1, 3–4, 6,
        7, 8–9
anti-inflammatory treatment of
        AD 97

antioxidant treatment of AD 96
antipsychotics
  atypical 25, 28
  depot formulations 30–1
  intravenous/intramuscular
      application 31
  mania 16, 17, 19
  OCD 74
  PTSD 64–5
  psychotic symptoms in
      dementia 100–1
  schizophrenia 25, 28–31
  switching between 29
anxiety in AD patients 100
aspirin *83*

benzodiazepines
  anxiety symptoms in AD 100
  mania 16
  panic disorder 41, 42
  social anxiety 53–4
  unipolar depression 4
beta-blockers 51
bipolar disorder 13–23
  augmentation of treatment
      17–18
  diagnostic criteria, mania
      *14–15*
  experimental approaches to
      treatment 18
  lifetime prevalence 13
  long-term treatment 19
  mood stabilizers *15*
  switching medication 16–17
  treatment decisions
      summarized *20–1*
  treatment of choice 15–16
  treatment, other options 18

treatments for discussion 18
  *see also* unipolar depression:
      diagnostic criteria
bipolar spectrum disorders 13
buspirone 30, 53

carbamazepine *15*
citalopram 3
clomipramine (CMI)
  OCD 71, 74–5
  panic disorder 43
clonazepam
  OCD 75
  panic disorder 42
  social anxiety 53
clonidine 65
clozapine 29, 30
CMI *see* clomipramine
  (CMI)
co-dergocrine mesylate 98
cognitive behavioural therapy
  (CBT)
  OCD 69
  panic disorder 41
  PTSD 62
  social anxiety 51
comorbid depression
  AD 100
  panic disorder 41
  schizophrenia 30
  social anxiety 52
compensation neurosis 57
compulsions *70, 71*
cyproterone acetate 75–6

delusions
  AD 100
  schizophrenia *26, 27*

dementia
  diagnosis 85, *86–7*, 87
  free radicals in 96
  reversible/potentially curable
    causes 87
  unrecognized 87
  *see also* Alzheimer's disease
    (AD)
dementia with Lewy bodies
    (DLB) 87, 88, 100–1
depression *see* bipolar
    disorder; comorbid
    depression; unipolar
    depression
donepezil *83*, 92, 95
drug–drug interactions 7, 30
dual antidepressants 4

electroconvulsive therapy
    (ECT)
  bipolar depression 18
  OCD 75
  schizophrenia 31
  unipolar depression 7
escitalopram 3, 39, 51

fenfluramine 74
fluoxetine 3
fluvoxamine 3, 30
free radicals 96

gabapentin 54
galantamine *83*, 93
*Ginkgo biloba 83*, 98

hallucinations
  AD 100
  schizophrenia *26, 27*

imipramine 64
indomethacin *83*
inositol
  OCD 75
  PTSD 66

kinase inhibitors *83*

lamotrigine
  bipolar disorder *15*
  PTSD 64
light therapy 7
lithium
  bipolar disorder *15*, 16
  unipolar depression 6
L-tryptophan 74

mania *see* bipolar disorder
manic-depressive
    psychosis *see*
    bipolar disorder
MAOIs *see* monoamine
    oxidase inhibitors
    (MAOIs)
memantine *83*, 98
milnacipran 4
mirtazapine 4
moclobemide
  panic disorder 43
  social anxiety 53
monoamine oxidase
    inhibitors (MAOIs)
  combined with SSRIs 7
  panic disorder 43
  social anxiety 52
mood stabilizers
  bipolar disorder *15*
  panic disorder 43

nefazodone
  PTSD 62, 65
  unipolar depression 4
neurosurgery for OCD 76
nimodipine
  AD *83*, 98
  bipolar depression 18

obsessions *70*, *71*
obsessive-compulsive disorder
    (OCD) 69–79
  augmentation of treatment
    74–5
  comorbidity 73
  diagnostic criteria *70–1*
  experimental approaches to
    treatment 76
  long-term treatment 77
  prevalence 69
  switching medication 73–4
  treatment decisions
    summarized *72*
  treatment of choice 71, *72*
  treatment, other options 75
  treatments for discussion 75–6
oestrogen replacement therapy
    *83*, 97
ondansentron 54

panic attacks 35, *36*, *37*
panic disorder 35–45
  augmentation of treatment 42
  comorbidity 41
  development of *38*
  diagnostic criteria 35, *36–7*
  differential diagnosis *39*
  experimental approaches to
    treatment 43–4

long-term treatment 44
  switching medication 41–2
  treatment decisions
    summarized *40*
  treatment of choice 38, 39, *40*
  treatment, other options 43
  treatments for discussion 43
paroxetine 4, 44
performance anxiety 48, 51
phenelzine
  OCD 75
  PTSD 64
  social anxiety 52
physostigmine 92
pindolol
  panic disorder 43
  social anxiety 54
piracetam 98
post-traumatic stress disorder
    (PTSD) 57–67
  augmentation of treatment
    64–5
  characteristic features
    58, 61
  diagnostic criteria *59–61*
  experimental approaches to
    treatment 65–6
  long-term treatment 66
  prevalence 58
  risk factors 61
  switching of medication 62,
    64
  time course *61*
  treatment decisions
    summarized *63*
  treatment of choice 62
  treatment, other options 65
  treatment to be discussed 65

propranolol
  performance anxiety 51
  PTSD 65
protease inhibitors *83*
psychotherapy
  bipolar disorder 19
  schizophrenia 33
  unipolar depression 9
PTSD *see* post-traumatic stress
    disorder (PTSD)
public speaking, fear of 48

reboxetine 4
reversible inhibitors of
    monoamine oxidase
    (RIMAS)
  panic disorder 43
  social anxiety 53
risperidone 74
rituals *70, 71*
rivastigmine *83*, 92

St John's wort 7–8
schizophrenia 25–33
  augmentation of treatment
    29–30
  comorbidity 30
  diagnostic criteria *26–8*
  experimental approaches to
    treatment 31
  long-term treatment 31, 33
  prevalence 25
  switching medication 29
  treatment decisions
    summarized *32*
  treatment of choice 28–9
  treatment, other options 30–1
  treatments for discussion 31

screening instruments for
    dementia 87–8
seasonal affective disorder 7
selective noradrenaline reuptake
    inhibitors (SNRIs) 54
selective serotonin reuptake
    inhibitors (SSRIs)
  combined with irreversible
    MAOIs 7
  comorbid disorders in
    schizophrenia 30
  depression/anxiety symptoms
    in AD 100
  OCD 69, 71, 73–4
  panic disorder 39, 41
  PTSD 62
  social anxiety 51, 52, 53
  unipolar depression 3–4, 6, 7
selegeline 96
serotonin agonists 76
sertindole 25, 101
sertraline 4, 44
sleep deprivation (SD) in
    unipolar depression 8
sleep disturbances in AD 101
SNRIs *see* selective
    noradrenaline reuptake
    inhibitors (SNRIs)
social anxiety disorder 47–55
  augmentation of treatment 53
  comorbidity 48, 52
  diagnostic criteria *50*
  disability 47
  experimental approaches to
    treatment 54
  fears *50*
  long-term treatment 54–5
  prevalence 48

social anxiety disorder (*cont*)
  subtypes 48
  switching medication 52–3
  treatment decisions
      summarized *49*
  treatment of choice 51–2
  treatment, other options 53–4
  treatments for discussion 54
social phobia *see* social anxiety
    disorder
sodium valproate *15*
SSRIs *see* selective serotonin
    reuptake inhibitors (SSRIs)

tacrine 92
tau-protein 81, *83*
TCAs *see* tricyclic anti-
    depressants (TCAs)
tetracyclic antidepressants 4
thyroid hormone
  bipolar depression 17, 18
  unipolar depression 6
transcranial magnetic
    stimulation (TMS)
  bipolar depression 18
  PTSD 65
  unipolar depression 8
tranylcypromine 52
traumatic events 58, *59*, 61
tricyclic antidepressants (TCAs)
  panic disorder 43

PTSD 64
  unipolar depression 4
L-tryptophan 74

unipolar depression 1–11
  augmentation of treatment 6–7
  diagnostic criteria *2–3*
  experimental approaches to
      treatment 8
  lifetime prevalence 1
  long-term treatment 8–9
  switching medication 6
  treatment decisions
      summarized *5*
  treatment of choice 3–4, 6
  treatment, other options 7–8
  treatments for discussion 8

vagus nerve stimulation (VNS)
    in unipolar depression 8
valproic acid *15*, 16
venlafaxine
  dual mechanism of action 4
  PTSD 65
  social anxiety 52, 54
  unipolar depression 4
verapamil 18
vitamin E *83*, 96

zolpidem 101
zopiclone 101